WITHDRAWN

Sociology for Health Professionals

Lani Russell

D0166073

Los Angeles | London | New Delhi
Singapore | Washington DC

CUYAHOGA COMMUNITY COLLEGE
EASTERN CAMPUS LIBRARY

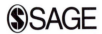

Los Angeles | London | New Delhi
Singapore | Washington DC

SAGE Publications Ltd
1 Oliver's Yard
55 City Road
London EC1Y 1SP

SAGE Publications Inc.
2455 Teller Road
Thousand Oaks, California 91320

SAGE Publications India Pvt Ltd
B 1/I 1 Mohan Cooperative Industrial Area
Mathura Road
New Delhi 110 044

SAGE Publications Asia-Pacific Pte Ltd
3 Church Street
#10-04 Samsung Hub
Singapore 049483

© Lani Russell 2014

First published 2014

Apart from any fair dealing for the purposes of research or private study, or criticism or review, as permitted under the Copyright, Designs and Patents Act, 1988, this publication may be reproduced, stored or transmitted in any form, or by any means, only with the prior permission in writing of the publishers, or in the case of reprographic reproduction, in accordance with the terms of licences issued by the Copyright Licensing Agency. Enquiries concerning reproduction outside those terms should be sent to the publishers.

Editor: Alison Poyner
Assistant editor: Emma Milman
Production editor: Katie Forsythe
Copyeditor: Clare Weaver
Proofreader: Imogen Roome
Indexer: Silvia Benvenuto
Marketing manager: Tamara Navaratnam
Cover design: Lisa Harper
Typeset by: C&M Digitals (P) Ltd, Chennai, India
Printed in Great Britain by Henry Ling Limited at
The Dorset Press, Dorchester, DT1 1HD

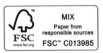

MIX
Paper from
responsible sources
FSC
www.fsc.org   FSC™ C013985

Library of Congress Control Number: 2013940228

British Library Cataloguing in Publication data

A catalogue record for this book is available from the British Library

ISBN 978-1-4462-5300-7
ISBN 978-1-4462-5301-4 (pbk)

CUYAHOGA COMMUNITY COLLEGE
EASTERN CAMPUS LIBRARY

Contents

List of figures and tables   vii
About the author   ix
Acknowledgements   x
Publisher's acknowledgements   xi
Companion website   xiii

Introduction   1

 1 Biomedicine   6
 2 Power   23
 3 Class   39
 4 Ethnicity   57
 5 Ageing   75
 6 Gender   91
 7 Sexuality   107
 8 Chronic illness and disability   122
 9 Mental health   140
10 Health care   155

Glossary   172
Key theorists   177
References   179
Index   201

List of figures and tables

Figures

1.1   Descartes' *Essai sur l'homme*   8
1.2   All Party Group on Muscular Dystrophy   18
      (Northern Ireland, 2012)
1.3   Biomedicine in Europe – key dates   20

2.1   Medicalization: At last! A cure!   31

3.1   Age-standardised mortality rates by seven-class   45
      NS-SEC for 2001–08, women aged 25–59
3.2   Adults aged 45–64 in routine and manual occupational   47
      groups are much more likely to have a limiting
      longstanding illness or disability than those from
      non-manual groups
3.3   Prevalence of Ischaemic Heart Disease (Heart Attack   48
      or Angina) or Stroke, by Social Class
3.4   *Shameless*   55

4.1   Image from J.C. Nott and George R. Gliddon (1854)   58
      Types of Mankind
4.2   Muslim Women's Sport Foundation Cobras, winners   67
      of the 2010 Futsal Festival, Kilburn
4.3   Prevalence of diabetes by mean BMI and sex in   68
      populations of West African origin

5.1   Images of older people in advertising material
      increasingly reflect social aspirations for healthy ageing   81

6.1   'Muff March' protest, December, 2011   101

7.1   Rejecting stigma. Demonstrators march in Durban,   117
       9 July 2000, on the first day of the XIII International
       AIDS Conference
7.2   Virtual sex: avatars   119

8.1   Mabel Cooper   133
8.2   Disabled activist outside the head office of the   135
       company Atos in London, 31 August 2012

9.1   'Ill' Patient, 'Well' Expert   146

10.1   Isaack Koedijck. Barber surgeon tending a peasant's   156
       foot (c. 1649–1650)
10.2   Interprofessional learning, Brown University,   166
       Providence, US

Tables

3.1   The Registrar General's Social Class classification   43
3.2   The National Statistics Socio-economic Classification   43
       system (NE-SEC)
3.3   Age standardised mortality (per 100,000 population)   46
       from selected causes within each social class group
       Men aged 20–59, Scotland 1990–1992

5.1   Percentage of respondents observing ageist activity   85

9.1   Percentage suffering from mental illness (England)   143

About the author

Lani Russell is a sociology lecturer in the Department of Social Sciences, Media and Journalism in the Glasgow School for Business and Society at Glasgow Caledonian University. Born in Australia, she studied at the University of Queensland and the University of Technology, Sydney, and worked at the Australian National University in Canberra before migrating to Brighton in 2000 and then to Glasgow the following year. At the University of Sussex she held a research fellowship working with Alistair Thomson and Jim Hammerton on a life history project collecting stories of post-war return migration to Australia. She later took up a second fellowship at Glasgow Caledonian University, conducting participatory action research with Pamela Abbott, Bill Hughes and Rachel Russell to promote race equality in the public sector. Since 2007 Lani has taught sociology of health and illness to large groups of students in all branches of nursing, midwifery, physiotherapy, podiatry, occupational therapy, radiography, diagnostic imaging, operating department practice and social work and is helping develop and deliver the new inter-professional practice framework in the School of Health. She leads the Honours module Ethnicity, Identity and Migration for the Social Science degree and her research interests focus particularly on ethnicity and migration, as well as health. Her paper about whiteness and diversity management was recently published online in *Ethnic and Racial Studies*.

Acknowledgements

For their excellent assistance at all stages of the writing process I thank Emma Milman and Alison Poyner in particular, and all the team at Sage. I am grateful for the warm support of my colleagues in the Sociology, History and Politics Subject Groups in my Department at Glasgow Caledonian University, especially Rachel Russell, Bill Hughes and Nancy Lombard. Several anonymous reviewers provided constructive feedback. Thank you to my students in the School of Health for their positivity and interest. For their love and enthusiasm, I am indebted to Roz Paterson, Wendy Russell, Jack Pezzey and Clare Russell and especially my parents, Mike and Elizabeth Russell, and partner, Honza Plášil.

Publisher's acknowledgements

Figure 1.1 is courtesy of Historical Collections & Services, Claude Moore Health Sciences Library, University of Virginia.

Figure 1.2 is republished with kind permission of the Muscular Dystrophy Campaign.

Figure 2.1 is republished with kind permission of www.cartonstock.com.

Figure 3.2 is courtesy of the authors and the University of Glasgow.

Table 3.3 Age standardised mortality (per 100,000 population) from selected causes within each social class group is republished by kind permission of Social and Public Health Sciences Unit, University of Glasgow.

Figure 3.4 is republished with kind permission of Matt Squire.

Figure 4.1 is from J.C. Nott and George R. Gliddon (1854) available at: http://museumvictoria.com.au/immigrationmuseum/discoverycentre/identity/people-like-them/the-white-picket-fence/timeline/

Figure 4.2 is republished with kind permission of the Muslim Women's Sport Foundation.

Figure 5.1 is courtesy of iStockphoto.

Figure 6.1 'Muff March' is from Alan Denney. Available at: www.flickr.com/photos/alandenney/6489281681/in/photolist-aTrgmV-aThKAp-aThKpK-aThKjV-aTEbAc-abd2f1/

Figure 7.1 is courtesy of Corbis Images.

Figure 7.2 is republished with kind permission of www.eddihaskell.com.

Figure 8.3 is courtesy of Corbis Images.

Figure 9.1 'Ill' Patient, 'Well' Expert is republished by kind permission of Catherine Pain. Copyright Open University. First appeared in *Society Matters*: www.open.ac.uk/platform/blogs/society-matters

Figure 10.3 is republished with permission of Mike Cohea and Brown University.

Reviewer acknowledgements

The publishers would like to extend their thanks to the following individuals for their invaluable feedback on the initial book proposal and draft chapters from the text:

Julie Bailey-McHale, University of Chester

Sabina Gerrard, University of Central Lancashire

Fiona Harris, University of Stirling

Karen Iley, University of Manchester

Dr Pam Lowe, Aston University

David Tait, Edinburgh Napier University

Karen Wild, Keele University

Companion website

Visit the companion website at www.sagepub.co.uk/russell to find a range of free teaching and learning resources for use in conjunction with this book.

For lecturers the website provides...

- **Teaching Resources** – ideas for using the **exercises** from the book in your teaching, plus **additional exercises** not included in the book – ideal for class-based discussion.
- **Overview for lecturers and teachers** – describes how the book and companion website resources can be used.

For students the website provides....

- **Video links** with the author's discussion to show how sociological concepts relate to real life situations.
- **Interactive self-test glossary of key terms** and **theorists** to help reinforce your learning.
- **Free journal articles** linked to each chapter to extend your learning and help you to reference a wider range of literature.

Introduction

So what is sociology anyway? A simple definition is that it is the systematic study of human beings in society. One way to begin to understand what sociology is about is to compare it with physiology or psychology. Physiology is interested in the biological aspects of human beings. In physiology you learn about the various organs of the body and how they work. In psychology, by contrast, you learn about the workings of the human mind. Like psychologists, sociologists seek to understand individual human beings. However, unlike psychologists, our starting point for doing this is way beyond the individual. Sociologists are interested in where individuals fit within 'big picture' patterns in society. For example, one of the most important achievements of sociologists of health and illness has been to map out the distribution of rich and poor people in society, to collect information about their health and then to show how a person's wealth makes a difference to their health. You will read more about this in Chapter 3.

So sociologists are interested in society and what patterns in society mean for the individual. This book talks often about 'social factors'. It is using the word 'social' in a slightly different way to the way that you may be most familiar with. You might talk about having a 'social life' or feeling 'anti-social'. In this sense, the word 'social' refers to relationships with other people. Sociologists also use the word 'social' to refer to relationships with other people but our focus is not only on people we may know or who might be in our immediate 'social circle'. For sociologists, 'social factors' refer not only to these 'close' relationships but to relationships between different groups of people on a very large scale. For example, you will never meet most of the other people who were born in the same year as you. There are too many of them. However, you have something in common with them. For example, if you were born in 1995 you probably grew up knowing what the internet is. People born in 1965 or 1935 did not. This makes people born in 1995 different to those older people. You may not feel as if you are in a group with everyone who was born the same year as you, but it can be very interesting and useful to think about patterns like this (more about that in Chapter 5). To use another example, your gender is something that connects you to everyone else of the same gender. People who share a gender have certain similarities in their lives, even though there may also be many differences between them (see Chapter 6). In the area of health and illness, sociologists have surveyed large groups of people to identify patterns in their health and illness. At what age do most people die? Why do people live longer in one country than in another? Why are suicide rates higher amongst young men than any other group? On average, when are most people at their most happy? By surveying large groups of people to answer these kinds of questions, sociologists can offer crucial information for governments and others which can be used to improve the lives of people.

An important aim of this book is to help you to begin to develop what has been referred to as a 'sociological imagination' (Wright Mills, 1959). We don't tend to see the 'big picture' when we think about our own lives day to day. We often experience obstacles and challenges as if they were ours alone. By considering trends and patterns across wider society, we can start to see individual problems from a different perspective. Here's an example:

I was recently referred for a scan of my uterus. I spent about ten minutes in the company of the radiographer who implemented the scan. During those ten minutes, whilst peering at the screen, she asked me: 'Do you have a family?' My first reaction to this question was confusion. I have two parents, a sister and brother-in-law, a niece, cousins, a partner. Yes, I have a family. In the next instant I realized that as she was looking at an image of my uterus, what the radiographer probably wanted to know was whether I had given birth to a child. 'No,' I said, 'I haven't had children'. I am sure the radiographer had no awareness of my confusion, and it would be exaggerating to say that she ruined my day. She did her job well and identified the source of the problems I'd been having. And because I am a sociologist I know that in England and Wales in 2011 20% of women born in the year that I was born did not have children (ONS, 2013a). I also know that the proportion of women who never have children is increasing (Parr, 2005). So I don't feel too bad about it! However, the radiographer did remind me – as I have been reminded in medical settings on other occasions – that some people who are married and have children assume that they are the only people with families. They may not be aware that many of us who don't live in conventional families don't like the presumption that our family is not a 'real' family.

This book does not cover every aspect of the sociology of health and illness. What it does aim to do, though, is to help you learn to stand outside of your own life and view things from a wider standpoint. I wrote the book because, having taught first-year students in health-related programmes at Glasgow Caledonian University for some years, I am aware that many new students feel a little daunted about learning sociology. While some students enjoy reading and thinking about new ideas, many of you are 'doers' who want knowledge that has application. Many of my students have decided to enter health and social care professions because they want to help people, not because they liked the idea of spending yet more years in the education system. The challenge for me and my team of tutors is to win over students who are not convinced that sociology is going to be worthwhile. That means working hard to present these ideas in a way that students can understand. Inevitably, as with any new learning, there are new words and jargon that can be discouraging for a beginner. I always say 'use a dictionary' but it can still be hard work to get to grips with the concepts. In addition, as I always explain in the first lecture, understanding sociology involves taking a conceptual leap. You need to change the way you have seen the world in the past. Some students, once they 'get' this, tell me it is pretty awesome. I thought it was awesome when I 'got' it. But a change like that can't happen overnight. You will need to spend time with the ideas, listening, reading, asking questions and trying to get your head around it. What I've tried to do when writing this book is to make your introduction to sociology as gentle and enjoyable as I can.

To facilitate that, each chapter contains the follow elements:

- Key issues – three short bullet points that tell you what the chapter is about
- Introduction
- 'Keywords' defined in boxes throughout the text
- Case studies – short examples to illustrate points made in the text
- Implications for practice – a short section outlining what the points made in the chapter mean for the day-to-day practice of health care professionals
- Summary – three bullet points summarizing the chapter
- Exercise – to help you actively develop your own understanding of the ideas in the chapter
- Further reading – a small number of introductory texts for students who wish to learn more about that topic

Most chapters also include a short history of the chapter topic around the beginning of the chapter. The reason for these small history lessons is to stimulate your imagination, to show you how much has changed. The geographical focus of the book is Britain. For reasons of length I have not tried to provide data from Scotland, Northern Ireland and Wales at every point. I also try to step back and provide a more global picture at various points. Throughout the book, links are made between chapters to help connect ideas that appear within more than one chapter. The book is designed so that you can read it cover to cover as the textbook for your course or you can dip into it and just read one chapter on its own. The following outline will give you an idea of the specific content of the ten chapters that follow:

Chapter 1 is on the topic of 'Biomedicine'. In our society, though we may not even think about this very much, we value a scientific approach to health problems. This is not the way most people in history thought about health. The scientific approach to health arose in Europe in the nineteenth century and is known as 'biomedicine'. By exploring biomedicine, and looking at some of the recent shifts in how we think about health, this chapter tries to stimulate your 'sociological imagination'.

Chapter 2 is about 'Power'. We do not usually think of people who work in health and social care as people who have power over others. However, the issue of power is very important for thinking about the ways in which wider society impacts on our health and on the work of health and social care practitioners. This chapter explores the idea that health care involves more than just caring for people. It takes place within unequal societies and reflects that wider context. 'Context' is a word you will read often in this book.

Chapter 3 considers 'Class'. Each of us has a place in the class structure of our society. Some have a very good position compared to others. They have more opportunities available to them and more resources to improve their lives. Others are disadvantaged in this respect. They may be unemployed, have a lower income and face many obstacles to improving their situation. This chapter shows that our position in society compared to others makes a major difference to our health. People who are worse off in general also tend to have worse health.

The subject of Chapter 4 is 'Ethnicity'. All of us belong to an ethnic group and have ideas about what it is that people from different groups have in common. This chapter explores these ideas about our differences and looks to history to understand why we think this way. It looks at some of the actual health differences that exist between ethnic groups and explores the reasons for those differences.

'Ageing' is the subject of Chapter 5. We think of ageing as a biological process but this chapter suggests that the process of ageing is not so automatic. The way that our society is organized and the way that we treat older people has a important impact on their health patterns.

Chapter 6 is about 'Gender'. It explores some of the differences between women and men which are not about biology but about the different lives, roles and ideas of men and women in our society. There are many health differences between men and women which reflect society, not just biology.

Chapter 7, 'Sexuality', considers how it is that we come to adopt our sexual identity, as 'gay' or 'straight', for example. It challenges the idea that there is a 'gay gene' and explores how attitudes about sexuality have changed over time in our society. It shows how people from sexual minorities have experienced unsatisfactory health and social care in Britain.

Chapter 8 explores 'Chronic illness and disability'. A growing proportion of people in society are suffering chronic illness. Both chronically ill and disabled people face a variety of physical challenges but this chapter shows the important ways that social organization and attitudes make a difference to their lives.

Chapter 9, 'Mental Health', considers why some people are less mentally healthy than others. What kind of factors make a difference to whether we are vulnerable to depression, anxiety or hearing voices? The chapter highlights the importance of social factors, particularly hardship and adversity.

The final chapter, Chapter 10, considers 'Health care'. Here, the job of being a health care professional is itself put under the microscope. This chapter is about some of the most important features of our health care system, how those features came about and what they mean for people working within the system.

At the end, you will find a long list of references which you can refer to if you wish to learn more. I hope you enjoy reading the book.

1

Biomedicine

Key issues

- The way we think about health and illness today reflects a way of thinking that dates back to the nineteenth century; it is known as the **biomedical model**
- The biomedical approach to health and illness has strengths but also weaknesses; it over-simplifies health problems in particular ways
- Health care practice today reflects the influence of the social and **biopsychosocial** models of health, which emphasize psychological and **social factors** influencing health and illness

Introduction

When you think about health care, what images come to mind? You may picture uniforms and sterile floors, white coats, plastic gloves and patients lined up in bed. It seems like 'common sense' to think about health in this way. However, this way of thinking about health is fairly recent. Our twenty-first century ideas about health can be traced back to the nineteenth century and the rise of an approach to human health that we now call 'biomedicine'. Looking at the early history of biomedicine can help us to stand back from our own experience of health and health care and think about what health means from a wider perspective.

> Biomedicine, biomedical model: an approach to health and illness which defines illness as the absence of disease, portraying the human organism as either functioning 'normally' or else dysfunctional and therefore diseased.

A Short History of Medicine

Our society still places great value on science and a scientific approach to problems, seen as rational, objective and unbiased. But for most of human history people did not aspire to being 'scientific'. In medieval Europe, life revolved around the church, and society was dominated by religious ideas. People believed that the source of knowledge was God. Knowledge should only be acquired through God's agents on earth, priests, who were morally equipped to interpret the word of God as expressed in the Bible. To tamper with nature was seen as immoral, because nature existed as it did because it was 'God's will'. Ideas about human health were situated within this framework. For example, people who had visual and auditory hallucinations and would today be diagnosed as suffering from schizophrenia were considered to be possessed by demons. Health care, for those who could afford it, was carried out by a variety of healers who might have quite different ideas about how to effect a cure (Elmer, 2004).

By the sixteenth and seventeenth centuries, European society was changing in a way that would affect the rest of the world. One person who was important in the development of new ideas was René Descartes (1596–1650), often referred to as the founder of modern philosophy. Descartes is significant in relation to health because he was the most important thinker to articulate clearly a view which suggested that the mind and the body are two separate spheres. He argued that the body could be seen as part of the physical world and the mind as part of the spiritual world (see Figure 1.1). The mind and body are connected, but separate. This idea was an important milestone on the road towards the development of modern medical ideas, or 'biomedicine'. The body was identified as the location for illness and part of the physical world. This was one step towards using scientific methods to try to understand how the body works and towards ending the former reluctance to interfere with the 'course of nature' (Seymour, 1998; Engel, 1977).

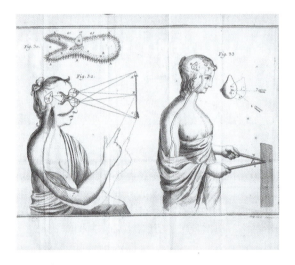

Figure 1.1   Note in Descartes' *Essai sur l'homme* the location of the soul, a teardrop shape inside the brain, seen as the controller of the body

Courtesy of Historical Collections & Services, Claude Moore Health Sciences Library, University of Virginia.

Descartes' ideas fitted with a new understanding of the world that would allow thinkers to engage in scientific experimentation without being labelled dangerous enemies of God. New social forces were emerging in society. These included manufacturers, small scale at first, who were increasingly motivated to develop new, faster and cheaper ways to produce things that would make them a profit in the marketplace. Over the course of several centuries, these new social forces became associated with enthusiasm for science and an intellectual movement now known as **the Enlightenment**. It is usually dated as starting in the late part of the seventeenth century and ending in 1800 at the beginning of the nineteenth century (you will read more about this in Chapters 2 and 3). Enlightenment thinkers celebrated 'reason' and rationality over superstition. They valued scientific methods of investigation – observation and experimentation – rather than religious authority. The following seventeenth-century text shows the influence of machine imagery in the views of early anatomists as they peered over corpses, trying to understand the workings of the human body:

> Whoever examines the bodily organism with attention will certainly not fail to discern pincers in the jaws and teeth: a container in the stomach: water-mains in the veins, the arteries and other ducts; a piston in the heart; sieves or filters in the bowels; in the lungs, bellows; in the muscles, the force of the lever; in the corner of the eye, a pulley, and so on. (Synnott, 1993: 23)

The Nineteenth-century Rise of Biomedicine

Biomedicine rapidly came to dominate approaches to health care over the course of the nineteenth century. This new scientific approach to health was associated with the rise of university medical training to ensure practitioners were experts in the science of medicine. Increasingly, the laboratory became the appropriate venue for medical research. The status of doctors and medical professionals increased as they formed their own organizations to set standards about who should and should not be allowed to practice health care (more about this in Chapter 10). As the medical establishment consolidated its influence in society, a variety of healers on the margins including herbalists and midwives were pushed aside (Lawrence, 1994; Brunton, 2004).

With the rise of biomedicine, patients' experience of medical care changed fundamentally. Where health care had been mainly carried out by traditional local healers at home, hospitals, places set aside especially for the treatment of the sick, now became the important site for health care (Jewson, 1976). In a society ever more focused on the idea of people as individuals, health care came to be about a relationship between two individuals: the medical expert, responsible for their individual conduct according to the standards of their profession, and the patient, responsible for monitoring their own health, reporting any problems and complying with the expert advice provided by the doctor (Gabe et al., 2004: 125).

Characteristics of Biomedicine

Biomedicine, the new scientific approach to medicine, was based on an underlying set of ideas about health that has been called 'the biomedical model'. That model rests on some key assumptions about the human body, health and illness. Four are discussed here.

The Body as a Machine

The simplest feature of the biomedical model is that it describes the body as if it were a machine. Anatomy was a particular interest in the nineteenth century, and there was great competition to obtain human bodies to dissect and study. The early doctors were enthusiastic to discover the mechanical way that the parts of the body work together. Consequently, an important characteristic of the biomedical model is to treat the body as a machine. Sarah Nettleton labelled this feature the '**mechanical metaphor**' (2006). The body is imagined in biomedicine as if it were a machine.

> Mechanical metaphor: a feature of the biomedical model of illness that portrays the human body as functioning essentially like a machine.

Mind-body Dualism

The biomedical model reflects the influence of the philosopher Descartes, mentioned earlier. Descartes was interested to understand the nature of human beings and consciousness and the relationship between the mind and the body. He suggested that we could distinguish between a person's brain and their mind, which are related, but not the same. Our ideas, beliefs and values cannot be reduced to biology, but belong to another realm. The body is governed by physical laws, but is also controlled by the mind (see Figure 1.1). This idea was essential for biomedicine to develop. However, it can also be associated with a view that emotions and beliefs – matters of the mind – were of secondary importance when it came to fixing body-machines (Seymour, 1998).

Discounting Emotion

The new scientific approach to health valued an objective, distanced approach to knowledge, against earlier approaches to knowledge, which were inconsistent, with individuals allowing their personal positions to influence how they understood the world. Against this, biomedicine was concerned to observe and survey the object of study in a disinterested way. From the perspective of the new medical experts, the opinion of the patient was just one of many factors which had to be disregarded when making a diagnosis. From a scientific point of view, the patient's opinion was of no value at all as the patient was likely to be biased about their own health. The focus was on understanding the workings of the body, governed by natural laws that do not differ across individuals. What this meant is that biomedicine tended to discount the ideas and opinions of the patient (Atkinson, 1988).

One Single Cause

Over the course of the nineteenth century medical experts became convinced that illness was something that started with a problem in a specific organ of the body. Then, their focus shifted to specific tissues. By the 1880s, attention had turned to organisms too small for the eye to see but capable of causing symptoms throughout the body, in particular, germs (Najman, 1980). The arrival of '**germ theory**', the idea that particular diseases could be explained by particular germs, marked the beginning of high-profile quests to identify crucial germs behind major diseases. It was hoped this would be the first step to finding a way to drive these germs from the body, using antitoxins or inoculation. The discovery of germs was credited with saving thousands of lives of people suffering from major killers of the time, diseases like smallpox, cholera, diphtheria and typhoid. It is not surprising, then, that the idea that all illness could ultimately be explained by a single cause became a key assumption of the biomedical model (Davis and George, 1993; Hart, 1985).

Germ theory: an explanation which identified micro-organisms as the essential agent for particular infectious diseases.

The Context for Challenges to the Biomedical Model

Through the course of the nineteenth century and into the twentieth, the influence and prestige of medicine as a science advanced steadily, as did science in general. New inventions and discoveries seemed to promise that science could solve many of humanity's problems. The Second World War, however, marked a point at which faith in science faltered. In particular, the 1945 bombing of Hiroshima, an act made possible by recent scientific advance, demonstrated that scientific progress could result in catastrophic destruction and loss of life.

Medical science also, despite its many achievements, began to deliver disappointments in the post-war years. Perhaps symbolic of this were the 12,000 babies born in the 1960s with shorter or missing limbs before the withdrawal of the morning sickness drug Thalidomide (Sargent, 2005: 240). The question of whether there would be a price to be paid for every cure found began to be asked. The 1960s also marked a time where people in countries across the world mobilized in a variety of social movements to confront governments whose authority had been called into question. One outcome of those movements was a cultural shift which saw populations become more politically aware and unwilling to accept the claims of elites claiming to act in their best interests.

In addition, the nature of illness changed. In the nineteenth century, germs were a major factor in morbidity and mortality. In that context a focus on finding the 'single cause' behind every illness made sense. However, from the mid-twentieth century, infectious disease became less important and the major causes of death were cancer and cardiovascular disease. Lifestyle and stress are now the most important threats to good health. Though childhood and infectious diseases remain major killers in the **majority world**, in the wealthiest countries today the major medical problems are chronic illnesses, conditions which have multiple causes (McKeown, 1979). As a consequence of all these social changes, after peaking in the 1950s the biomedical model began to be the target of increasing criticism. In recent decades biomedicine has been challenged from many quarters, including by a variety of health care professionals. As a result, conceptions of health and illness and health care practice have had to change (Wade and Halligan, 2004).

Majority world: a term used in preference to 'developing' or 'third world' countries, which attempts to avoid describing those countries in terms of how they appear from the viewpoint of those in the wealthiest countries.

Sociological Criticisms of Biomedicine

Sociologists in particular have been very critical of biomedicine. A sociologist is a social scientist who uses systematic methods to understand how the lives of individual people fit in with 'big picture' patterns in society – patterns of inequality, for example (more about that in Chapter 3). In recent decades, sociologists and some health professionals have argued forcefully that the biomedical model has some fundamental weaknesses. Any model is an oversimplification of reality we use to help us think about something complex. The danger is that by reducing complex processes to simple ones a model may *mis*-represent reality.

The metaphor of the body as a machine, for example, though very useful, oversimplifies reality. If the body is treated as a machine the focus is on physical symptoms that can be observed. Symptoms are seen as the signal that a breakdown has occurred in the body machine. The implication is that to treat illness it is necessary to examine the machine with the aim of removing the symptom. However, one problem with this approach is that removing the symptom may not solve the problem; an underlying illness might still be present. Another problem is that when trying to fix the problem, the biomedical approach focuses on the body itself. The idea that the breakdown may have to do with something outside the person does not fit with this model. As will be argued throughout this book, external factors outside the human body such as pollution, bad housing, dangerous neighbourhoods, domestic abuse and inadequate food and water supplies can all have a major impact on a person's health, but the 'body as machine' approach does not consider such factors (Nettleton, 2006).

As suggested above, the biomedical model can be criticized for arguing that all illness can be explained in relation to a single cause. Modern illnesses associated with stress and lifestyle factors do not have a single cause. Even diseases that are caused by germs need particular conditions in which to thrive. It is also the case that some health conditions do not necessarily cause any symptoms. People who have the Human Immunodeficiency Virus (HIV) or high blood pressure may not be ill. The opposite is also true – it is possible to have symptoms without having a recognizable health condition. People who suffer from conditions like Chronic Fatigue Syndrome (CFS) or Myoencephalitis (ME), for example, have struggled to have these syndromes accepted as diseases. In each of these examples, the idea that any illness must have symptoms stemming from a single cause is an obstacle to maximizing human health (Nettleton, 2006).

We also now know that the race to discover relevant germs and highly publicized 'medical breakthroughs' in the nineteenth century were not the most important factors in the success of the battle against tuberculosis and other diseases. Indeed, most of the drugs developed in this period would by today's standards be considered ineffective (Fitzpatrick, 2008: 9). The more important but less glamorous achievement of biomedical research at that time was to highlight the potential for germs to be spread through unclean water. This recognition led to the provision of cleaner water supplies, resulting in dramatic increases in life expectancy (McKeown, 1979; Szreter, 1988).

This is a lesson about biomedicine that is still relevant today. Worldwide, simple poverty continues to be the most important health hazard. Measles and tuberculosis are still major killers in the majority world and fatality rates are high amongst the very young because malnutrition has weakened their ability to fight the disease. Chapter 3 will present evidence that shows that in developed countries a person's degree of wealth or poverty also has a significant impact on their health. Too often, biomedical problems have been assumed to have biomedical causes and solutions, when the answers lie beyond the scope of individual practitioners.

Sociologists argue that all illness is socially constructed. How we understand our health or illness is a product of the society we live in. This does not mean that illness is not real, but that we can never understand bodily experiences such as illness except through the medium of our culture. Biomedical experts, however, have tended not to see it that way. The suggestion that biomedicine might reflect a historically situated approach to understanding health and illness rather than a purely objective standpoint is challenging for some scientists. One consequence of denying the social construction of illness is that medical professionals may fail to recognize ways in which their ideas about health and illness reflect social values (Lupton, 2012).

For example, in the nineteenth century doctors played an important role in ensuring that women were prevented from entering higher education. They argued that women's biological inferiority mean that women should confine themselves to the domestic sphere. Entering higher education was simply physiologically dangerous for women and could only lead to physical or mental breakdown (Talairach-Vielmas, 2007) (you can read more about biomedicine and women's health in Chapter 6). Today it seems obvious that these doctors (all men) were wrong. Their socially inherited views about the appropriate place for women in society influenced the way they interpreted the physiological evidence. Moreover, the history of social values influencing medical ideas about normality and abnormality is a history that is still continuing. As values change, future criticism of current ways of thinking about what is 'normal' and 'abnormal' is inevitable.

The Social and Biopsychosocial Models of Health

In response to the various limitations of biomedicine already discussed, attempts have been made to devise a new model for health and illness, one that retains what is most useful in biomedicine but addresses some of its weaknesses. Today we can talk about the social model (Morgan et al., 1985), or the biopsychosocial model, a model conceptualized by the psychiatrist George Engel. Working every day with people struggling with psychiatric problems, the psychiatrist George Engel was particularly aware that there was a problem with the idea that the mind and the body should be considered separately. Engel argued that the boundaries between health and illness are not clear because both ideas are influenced by cultural, social and psychological considerations. The job of the psychiatrist, Engel argued, should be to weigh up what balance of social, psychological and biological factors have led to the person feeling unwell or having a problem functioning as they think they should. A biopsychosocial model, he argued, would recognize that it is the physician's role to accept responsibility to evaluate whatever problem the patient presents and recommend a course of action. The focus of this biopsychosocial practice would be not just a body in need of repair but a thinking, feeling, social being, that is, a being with a biological, a psychological and a social self (Engel, 1977).

> Biopsychosocial model: an approach to health and illness which sees illness as reflecting psychological and social as well as biological factors.

In what ways is the self social? The social model of health emphasizes in particular the role of wider society in how we experience and understand health issues. The social model of health emphasizes the multiple roots of health issues and the diverse possibilities for achieving health outcomes. For example, we think about the impact on a person's health of their class, their gender, their age, ethnicity, any disabilities they have and their sexuality. Social factors include issues such as poverty and housing which form an essential part of the wider context in which biological processes take place. In addition, social factors refer not only to our interactions with people close to us (our 'social life', as it is informally known) but to our indirect engagement with **norms** and values shared by people we have not met and groups which we may only vaguely be aware of being part of. These norms and values make up the culture of our society. Our ideas about what is and what isn't a medical problem are ideas we learn in the context of our society and those ideas have implications for health care.

> Social factors: factors which affect an individual and involve other people, including the many people to whose lives we are indirectly connected even though we may never have met them (for example, wider social groups to which we are connected such as our class, gender, ethnic group, sexuality and nation).
>
> Norms: informal understandings amongst groups of people about the right way to behave.

It is also useful to think of some health issues as psychosocial. There are particular events and experiences in our society which put stress on human beings and our ability to cope. Sociological studies have explored, for example, adverse affects on health produced by socio-cultural instability, rapid social change, being isolated or struggling to make ends meet (Marmot and Wilkinson, 2009). This concept will be explored again in Chapter 3 and in other chapters of this book. It is easy to see what can happen if medical experts do not have an awareness of these kinds of factors. Imagine, for example, a person who has unexplained physical symptoms which are associated with ongoing abuse or alcoholism. If these factors are not recognized, a traditional biomedical response might be to prescribe the patient pain killers or some other kind of medication, a strategy which may only lead to new problems and does not go to the main cause of the problem anyway (see Case Study: Women's Chronic Pelvic Pain).

> Psychosocial factors: social experiences and environments which cause stress for individuals, making them more vulnerable to illness.

Women's Chronic Pelvic Pain: Not Just a Bodily Problem

Chronic pelvic pain (CPP) affects about 4% of women in developed countries, making it quite a common illness, but one which is not easily addressed. Researchers in Brazil suggest that an important part of the problem is a biomedical focus on the part of most health professionals. CPP is not just a physiological problem. It also impairs a woman's social, professional, marital and maternal life. It may lead to job loss, divorce, limited social contact and reduced physical activity. A woman's ability to cope depends on meanings, beliefs and values, not only on her physical state. Women with CPP say that they struggle to plan their daily lives because of the constant threat of pain. Yet they are also overwhelmingly concerned with finding out the main 'cause' of their pain, partly because they wish to establish the legitimacy of their symptoms and avoid being labelled as 'crazy' or 'neurotic'. Evidence suggests CPP is complex and has many causes, but health care professionals may also be overly focused on finding a single 'cause' for the illness. They may even add to the distress of women with CPP by becoming preoccupied with distinguishing between 'real' and 'psychological' pain, despite evidence that any line between the two is hazy. Emphasis on hormones, menstruation or menopause may also be associated with suggestions that pain is a normal part of being female, implying CPP pain is unavoidable and must simply be endured. By focusing on the biomedical aspects of this problem, professionals neglect the social context, ideas and feelings of sufferers, adding to their feelings of impotence and frustration.

Source: Souza, P.P., Romão, A.S., Rosa-e-Silva, J.C., Reis, F.C., Nogueira, A.A. and Poli-Neto, O.B. (2011) 'Qualitative research as the basis for a biopsychosocial approach to women with chronic pelvic pain', *Journal of Psychosomatic Obstetrics and Gynecology*, 32(4): 165–72.

The social model of health focuses on prevention, not only cure. It stresses the ability of the individual or **lay person** to make healthy choices and find healthy spaces in which to live. This approach has been described as salutogenic, as distinct from the biomedical approach which is pathogenic, focused on the discovery of the relevant pathogen. According to this model, health care is not only about curing people but about supporting them to maintain their health or achieve rehabilitation. If we focus on lifestyle and stress as causes of ill health, rather than solely on germs, health care becomes about being supported to manage our wider environment, the place where we live, and our social relationships (Becker et al., 2010).

Lay person: a person who is not an expert in a particular area.

Salutogenesis: an approach to health and illness which focuses on factors that support human health rather than those which foster disease.

The Rise of Lay Involvement in Health Care

The move towards a social model of health care is also associated with the rise of lay involvement in health care. Today in the field of health it is recognized that the boundary between the experts and the non-experts is not the high wall it once was. Many lay people today have acquired at school or through the media or their own investigations some of the biomedical knowledge that medical professionals encounter at university. Many people with long-term health conditions, in particular, have become highly educated and perhaps also politically active about their condition (see Figure 1.2). Lay people have also become consumers of health who can and do 'shop around'. If they are not happy with what is available they may seek alternatives, and these alternatives may be in fields which have traditionally been

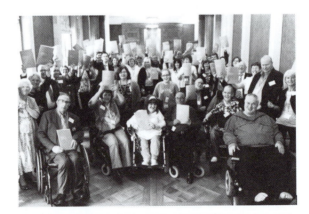

Figure 1.2 Supporters at the launch of the McCollum Report by the All Party Group on Muscular Dystrophy (Northern Ireland, 2012)

Photograph courtesy Muscular Dystrophy Campaign

on the margins of acceptability from the point of view of medical professionals. Some of these alternatives are even beginning to be institutionalized such as osteopathy, acupuncture and homeopathy (Saks, 2006).

New Approaches to Health

New approaches to health have arisen which reflect lay involvement in health care and recognition of the importance of social factors. Government health policy today recognizes the need to address health inequalities by redressing poverty and targeting cultural and lifestyle issues with health implications, for example unhealthy habits such as smoking and poor diets. Central to these approaches is the empowerment of lay people. Because lay people are more knowledgeable, medicine is becoming less mysterious and inaccessible. This has implications for health care practice. Different people have different ideas about what good health means, so a health professional needs to be able to communicate with a client about their own understanding of their health so they can work with them and perhaps negotiate with them if they are resistant to professional advice. Taking account of how people feel and how they understand their own health situation has increasingly become part of mainstream medicine (White, 2005).

Health is no longer about 'doctor knows best' but is implicated in the judgements that people make, with the help of experts, about lifestyle and risk. So 'therapy', once something done by a medical expert to a patient, becomes something which is implicated in the everyday lives of non-experts. There is a strong implication in this of our health becoming our responsibility. It can be argued that approaches to health care are now becoming more pluralistic, with some resemblance to the situation that existed in the eighteenth century prior to the rise of biomedicine. A variety of different and competing medical practices based on different health beliefs now co-exist.

The proliferation of alternative healing systems and different ideas about what is therapeutic has meant that those working from a purely biomedical model have had to rework that model to some extent to accommodate the variety of healing systems, beliefs and knowledge that are now widely available in the therapeutic market place (see Case Study: Attitudes to Complementary and Alternative Medicine (CAM)). Biomedicine has had to change and to shift its model of health, health care and illness to survive and continue to prosper in a world that has become more sceptical about its value and worth (White, 2005). Discussion about the extent to which biomedical ways of thinking still dominate the practice of medicine today is ongoing.

Although biomedicine is still the model that dominates medical theory and practice, it has lost ground to a more holistic approach (Smith et al., 2013). Figure 1.3 shows some of the key dates in these developments over time.

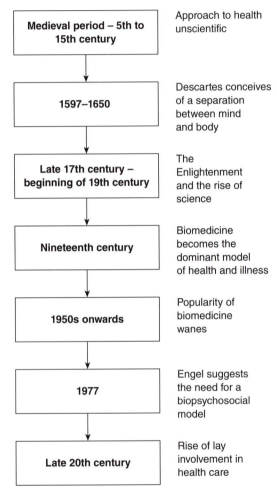

Figure 1.3   Biomedicine in Europe – key dates

CASE STUDY

Attitudes to Complementary and Alternative Medicine (CAM)

Researchers in Galway, Ireland were interested to know more about CAM use, given its growing popularity. They surveyed 219 cancer patients, 301 non-cancer hospital volunteers and 156 health care professionals, including doctors, nurses, physiotherapists, pharmacists, speech and language, and occupational therapists, all involved in the care of cancer patients. The survey found that one in three had used CAM, mostly natural supplements like probiotics or fish oil, vitamins, green tea and herbal or folk remedies. Massage therapy, acupuncture, yoga and chiropractic therapy were also popular. However, only one in three users voluntarily reported CAM use to their doctors. Most of those who did not mention CAM use said it was because the doctor never asked (34.6%) or because they thought that the doctor would not understand or would disapprove (9.6%).

Interestingly, the survey found health care professionals were more likely to use CAM than others surveyed, including 80% of pharmacists, 49.2% of nurses and 37% of physiotherapists, but only 28.8% of doctors. Eighty per cent of professionals felt they were not up to date with the best evidence on CAM use. This is important because, despite the benefits of many CAMs, some CAM ingredients can have negative effects for cancer sufferers. Shark cartilage, for example, has been shown to have no effect on tumour growth but causes severe gastrointestinal toxicity and the herb St John's Wort reduces the effectiveness of chemotherapy. The researchers concluded by recommending provision of CAM training for health care professionals at university, now introduced in several countries.

Source: Chang, K.H., Brodie, R., Choong, M.A., Sweeney, K.J. and Kerin, M.J. (2011) 'Complementary and alternative medicine use in oncology: a questionnaire survey of patients and health care professionals', *BMC Cancer*, 11(196).

•••

Implications for Practice

A biopsychosocial approach has been promoted particularly in recent years in relation to chronic conditions such as musculoskeletal conditions, rheumatoid arthritis and chronic pain, where the importance of work patterns as well as physiological and psychological factors is well supported. The biopsychosocial model has been embraced by particular professions such as nursing and, more recently, occupational therapy and physiotherapy (Sanders et al., 2013; Ryan and Carr, 2010). In other professions which may involve brief and limited contact with service users, focus on physiological problems may mean that psychological and social factors seem of lesser importance. However, it is important to recognize that all service users work to improve their health in the context of the particular circumstances of their own life and within a society that offers particular ways of thinking about health. As the following chapters will explore further, these social factors have crucial implications for health, making a biopsychosocial approach essential.

Summary

- The traditional biomedical model started from an understanding of the body as a machine; issues to do with the mind were secondary
- A sociological approach to health and illness recognizes that a person's health must be understood in the context of their wider social environment
- Health care practice today involves considering not only the biological aspects of a person's wellbeing but social and psychosocial factors as well

Exercise

Think of the profession you are training for now. For a moment, think of the body as a machine, and yourself as the mechanic. List some of the 'repairs' your service users might need. Now, remind yourself of some of the social and psychosocial factors mentioned in this chapter. How would taking these kinds of factors into account change the way you approach the job of helping people who need 'repairs'?

Further Reading

Lupton, D. (2012) *Medicine as Culture: Illness, Disease and the Body in Western Societies*. Third edition. London: Sage.

Porter, R. (2004) *Blood and Guts. A Short History of Medicine*. London: Penguin.

 Online readings

To access further resources related to this chapter, visit the companion website at www.sagepub.co.uk/russell

Adams, J., Braun, V. and McCreanor, T. (2012) 'Gay men talking about health: are sexuality and health interlinked?', *American Journal of Men's Health* 6(3): 182–93.

2

Power

Key issues

- The work of health professionals reflects powerful groups and ideas in society
- Medical communities are associated with changing ideas in society about the parameters of health
- Changing conceptions of health are also maintained and developed in the thoughts, conversations and routines of lay people

Introduction

In all our lives, there are people who have power over us. Some of these people are close to us, people we see regularly – our boss, landlord or parent, for example. Others, such as the Prime Minister or the Vice-Chancellor of our university, are more distant. What all of these people have in common is that they are in a position in relation to us which means that they may require us to behave in particular ways – and we will mostly obey. Social **power,** that is, power between people, can be simply defined as our ability to control the behaviour and perhaps also the viewpoint of others.

Power: a capacity to dominate in relation to the actions or ideas of other people.

The issue of power has been of great interest to sociologists studying health and illness. Your first thought may be that power is not very important in relation to medicine. People usually only visit a health care professional of their own free will. They can choose to accept or reject the advice given to them. Nonetheless, issues of power are very important to understanding the nature of the relationship between a health care professional and a **lay person**. In Chapter 1 it was suggested that biomedicine is presented as being dispassionate and neutral but that in practice, health care has reflected particular views and interests. This chapter considers some of the ways questions of power arise in relation to health care.

Medical Power: The Power of Authority

To understand power, it is useful to start by considering groups who have been granted official sanction to punish those who do not comply, such as the police or the army. Ultimately, this type of social power rests on the right and potential to use force. Yet day to day, even the police and the army do not usually have to use force. In the same way that a teacher knows their ability to punish is not enough to keep control in a classroom, members of the police and the army know an important aspect of their power is authority. The extent to which they can control a situation depends on whether their intervention is seen as legitimate, whether it is accepted as just and right (Gramsci, 1971). Health professionals can be said to have power, but is power that is based on authority (Friedson, 1975; Macdonald, 1995). In particular, our willingness to obey a medical professional rests on whether we are convinced of their expertise. If we were uncertain that our medical helper had completed the appropriate university degree, for example, we might be less willing to follow their directions. This issue about the authority of health care professionals will be explored further in Chapter 10: Health Care.

The Sick Role

To think about medical authority as a kind of power is a challenge to the idea that the job of making a medical diagnosis is mainly or essentially a scientific matter. The role of the GP is not purely determined by the scientific facts they find in front of them. The doctor performs their role knowing that 'society' has certain expectations of them. Their task is to dispense medical help, but it is also to do it in such a way as to reinforce social values. As suggested in Chapter 1, it is important to remember that 'social' in this context does not refer simply to our relationships with friends and other people in our lives, though that is one aspect of what sociologists mean when they use the term 'social'. Throughout this book **social factors** refer to factors that reflect wider society. That is, not just the people we know but the many people whose lives we are indirectly connected to even though we may never have met them. For example, there is an expectation in modern society that a person in employment has a responsibility to look after their own health so that they can attend work. This is a 'social' value and it is reinforced by doctors. Sickness is usually thought of as a condition determined by our bodies. However, it is also a condition that reflects society. Whether a person is designated 'sick' depends on social, not biological rules.

One way to understand this is to recognize that when a person is diagnosed as being sick by a doctor, they take on a kind of social role. The theorist Talcott Parsons (1950) called this social role the 'sick role'. To say that sickness is a social role means that there are unspoken rules and norms of behaviour that go with being sick. When a doctor agrees that a person is sick, they are automatically granted certain rights but also responsibilities. The person now has a right to stay home from university or work while they are unwell. They have a right to care from a qualified medical practitioner. However, they also have a responsibility to follow the advice of their GP and try to overcome the illness quickly; it is assumed that this special status as a 'sick' person will only be temporary.

The effect of the sick role is to make GPs gatekeepers who police and regulate who is seen as sick and who is seen as well. It has been suggested that if this sick role did not exist, people would be able to make their own judgement about whether they were well enough to work or study, and as a whole we would be less productive, and that this would be bad for everyone. From this perspective the sick role reinforces the value of work in our society and is seen as being 'functional' for society (Parsons, 1950). Critics, however, have suggested that the sick role is not good for everyone in society. Being diagnosed as ill, for example, may result in hospitalization, which can be dehumanizing and change a person's life so much that they find it very difficult to go back to being a 'healthy' person again (Goffman, 1961).

Medicine and Capital

The idea of the sick role highlights the social aspects of health care and the role that health care might play in reinforcing dominant values in society. Health care, from this perspective, can be seen as involving '**social control**'. One very influential approach to questions of social control and power comes from the radical nineteenth-century German philosopher, Karl Marx. From the point of view of Marxist sociologists, the role played by health care professionals in society needs to be understood by starting from a recognition of global inequality, both in terms of power and wealth (Navarro, 1976).

> Social control: processes in society that ensure people follow the formal and informal rules of society.

As discussed in Chapter 1, the movement of ideas called **the Enlightenment,** brought science to the problems of human health; the result was **biomedicine**. In Chapter 1 it was implied that there were positives and negatives to this development. The Enlightenment preceded, and was associated with, the development of **capitalism** (more about that in Chapter 3). This new economic system brought about an expansion of industry as new businesses competed to make profit. It also led, indirectly, to the development of a public health system. As mines and factories developed and expanded, the powerful men who owned these enterprises soon noticed that workers who were constantly ill and died young, as they did during the industrial revolution, disrupted business. In addition, from the nineteenth century onwards, working people themselves pressured governments to introduce legislation to protect them and provide affordable health care.

Capitalism: a society in which ownership and control of production and business for profit in a competitive economy is the most important means of access to wealth and power.

Today, from a neo-Marxist perspective, the concentration of wealth in a small number of hands and the organization of production around competition for profit has been responsible for new health problems. In the **majority world**, large proportions of national income go to paying interest on international loans, perpetuating a cycle of disadvantage which breeds ill health. Poverty and malnutrition are major factors in global ill health. Being poor, for example, is a major risk factor for cardiovascular or heart disease, the disease which kills the most people in the world in both rich and poor countries (more about poverty and health in Chapter 3). In addition to cardiovascular disease, leading causes of death are lung infections and other infectious diseases like HIV/AIDS, tuberculosis, diarrhoeal diseases and malaria as well as complications of pregnancy and childbirth. All of these diseases are linked directly to poverty through factors like unclean water and sanitation and malnutrition (Benatar et al., 2011).

In addition, as Marxists have highlighted, private companies are directly involved in making large sums of money from health care. These include those companies that provide medical services and technology, as well as the powerful pharmaceutical industry, medical insurers and legal firms that represent patients suing practitioners for medical malpractice. In Britain, private companies commissioned to build hospitals and other facilities for the NHS have received billions of pounds from the government and will continue to receive large sums as interest for decades (Pollock, 2010).

Finally, Marxist and neo-Marxist analyses also emphasize ways the economic system benefits wealthy elites indirectly. For example, the focus of the health care system is on the individual. Information is provided by GPs and other health care professionals to individuals who are charged with taking responsibility for their own treatment. This focus on the individual, however, obscures the nature of our social reality. It gives the impression that health problems are the result of the actions of individuals and so hides the importance of inequality and the role played by the beneficiaries of inequality (Navarro, 1976; Crawford, 2008).

Sick Because of Health Care?

Marxists draw attention to the ways that our unequal society breeds ill health and ways health care itself benefits wealthy elites. Others suggested that modern health care has also changed the very way we experience and think about our own health and attempt to heal ourselves. By this view, medicine can be seen as invading our individual liberty in a fundamental way. Ivan Illich was a radical priest whose important book, *Limits to Medicine* (1976), made the provocative argument that health care had become an obstacle to good health. In particular, Illich argued that our society is characterized by **'iatrogenesis'**, which literally means, medical intervention which, instead of curing, actually *causes* illness.

> Iatrogenesis: medical intervention which, instead of curing, actually causes illness.

One obvious type of iatrogenesis is where medicine has undesirable side effects. By the twenty-first century, instances of people coming to unintended harm as a result of seeking medical help had become a major issue. In England and Wales in 2011, for example, 2,950 people died in patient safety incidents (where an unintended or unexpected incident resulted in patient harm in NHS-funded health care) with 92,780 people suffering moderate or severe harm (NRLS, 2013). It is now widely accepted that antibiotics, celebrated in the 1940s as opening a new era in health care, had the unintended consequence of stimulating the development of highly resistant and therefore more dangerous micro-organisms (Davies and Davies, 2010). The rise of the powerful pharmaceutical industry has resulted in far-reaching prescription of drugs for a variety of conditions, many of those drugs causing addiction, sleeping difficulties or personality changes (Law, 2006).

In all of these examples, medical intervention has resulted in unexpected negative clinical outcomes. Illich argued, however, that there are also negative outcomes from health care which relate to our capacity for self-care. 'Medically sponsored behaviour', he wrote 'restricts the vital autonomy of people by undermining their competence in growing up, caring for each other and ageing' (Illich, 1976: 15). Biomedicine has provided us with an ever-expanding set of new technologies and treatments to combat our health problems. However, one consequence of this is that people are more and more reliant on the medical profession to provide them with a solution. We expect to be provided with a treatment even in situations where it would be better to change our environment or simply do nothing.

More importantly, the more we rely on medical experts for diagnosis, the less ability we will have to self-diagnose, to decide ourselves what is wrong with us. Our reliance on medicine means we look for medical solutions to our problems at the expense of more traditional, intuitive approaches to our health (Hindley and Thomson, 2005; Sennett, 2008). A medical diagnosis may be more scientific but it may also be an alternative to a non-medical approach which may be more appropriate. For example, when someone is dying, a medical approach focused on alleviating symptoms is not actually offering any help with the main challenge they face, which is how to prepare for death (for more on death and dying, see Chapter 5). The arguments Illich made suggest an important aspect of power in relation to health care. Power can relate the ability to influence others to behave in particular ways, but power is also about knowledge. An important aspect of power is the ability to influences others to see things from a particular perspective.

Medicalization

When Parsons noted the social role played by the health care professional when providing a diagnosis (the 'sick role'), he saw this as an essentially positive feature of our society. The health care professional is a trustworthy gatekeeper, safeguarding the social values of society for the good of all. Others have highlighted how medical diagnoses may result in negative outcomes, both for patients and for society. Writing in 1975, the theorist Irving Zola gave the example of contraception:

> The physician while dispensing birth control information often functions in a moral capacity. Personal experience, as well as the literature of female liberation, is replete with cases of young single women being lectured, chastised, ridiculed, embarrassed and even refused help or a referral when they approach a physician for the pill, an IUD or a diaphragm. (1975: 84)

The technology of birth control has obviously improved a little since Zola's day, but this description of women feeling judged in a health care setting does not seem so strange, even nearly 40 years later. Zola argued that health care is always socially involved and for that reason it is impossible to separate medical judgements from social, political and moral judgements (Zola, 1972). Traditionally, moral authority is a quality more associated with judges, teachers or religious figures. However, in their day-to-day work health care professionals are in a position to advise people on what is correct and good behaviour. Medical experts have been influential in shaping our moral attitudes to issues such as sexual conduct, abortion, access to IVF technology and euthanasia (Lupton, 2012).

In addition to informing ideas about what is normal and good, the medical community is in a special position to contribute to the re-working of understandings of social problems. **Medicalization,** an idea pioneered by Zola and Illich, refers to a process by which issues in society come to be thought of and understood in a medical way. A whole range of issues and problems have – particularly over the last 150 years – come to be defined in medical terms (see Figure 2.1). For example, for several centuries up to the nineteenth century, women who refused to eat were regarded as holy, as demonstrating their piety or spiritual purity. In 1874 Dr William Gull coined the term 'anorexia nervosa'. With this category, Gull medicalized self-starvation. Since then we have come to understand food avoidance in terms defined by medical discourse (Griffin and Berry, 2003).

> Medicalization: a process by which previously non-medical issues in society come to be thought of and understood in a medical way.

Another aspect of life which has been medicalized is childbirth. From occurring in the home, with the help of family and a neighbourhood midwife, with little equipment or drugs, and at whatever pace the birth happened to take place, the whole experience of childbirth was changed with the rise of biomedicine. Labour was relocated to a hospital setting, and untrained midwives were marginalized as university-educated men began to take control of the birth process. A growing array of technologies and techniques transformed the experience of childbirth: scans, foetal monitors, caesareans, pain-killers and epidurals. One consequence of this medicalization has been that many women's lives have been saved where otherwise they would have died in childbirth. Many agree, however, that this benefit also came at a cost in relation to women's control over the birthing process. Medicalization of childbirth made women reliant on (predominantly male) medical experts (Oakley, 1980).

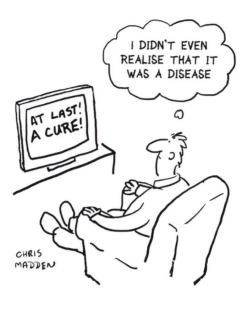

Figure 2.1   Medicalization: At last! A cure!

Source: www.cartoonstock.com

A more recent example of medicalization is hyperactivity. Fifty years ago, children who behaved badly were seen as naughty. Today, as a result of a process of medicalization in society, their behaviour may be understood in terms of the disease category known as hyperkinetic syndrome. They may very commonly receive a diagnosis of Attention Deficit Hyperactivity Disorder (ADHD) for which the drug Ritalin is now widely prescribed (Rafalovich, 2013). Other problems or aspects of life which have been medicalized in recent decades include insomnia, sadness, shyness, sexuality, drinking, baldness, hairiness, body shape, teenage misbehaviour, restless legs, eating at night, learning disabilities and sexual dissatisfaction (see Case Study: Orgasm Inc.).

Orgasm Inc: The Medicalization of Female Sexual Dysfunction

In the twenty-first century, pharmaceutical companies inspired by the financial success of Viagra are working to produce a female equivalent. Conferences have been held and diagnostic tools devised to explore and 'educate' the public about a

(Continued)

CASE STUDY

(Continued)

problem they now claim is widespread: female sexual dysfunction (FSD). Ideas about what exactly this problem involves (a problem with the vagina, with hormones or with brain chemicals) have changed as different types of drugs have been considered as potential 'cures' by the industry (Moynihan, 2010: 341). Companies quoted widely a 1999 claim that 43% of women suffer from sexual dysfunction. Yet this figure was soon discredited, and one of the lead academics who produced the original 43% figure has stated that statistic was not meant to represent the percentage of women with a treatable condition. Other research suggests that lack of interest in sex amongst women is often a result of stress or relationship difficulties, is not in itself considered a serious issue by most women and a medical solution is therefore inappropriate. The New View are activists lobbying against the misrepresentation of female sexuality by the pharmaceutical industry campaign (www.fsd-alert.org). See also orgasminc.org.

Sources: Moynihan, R. (2010) 'Merging of marketing and medical science: female sexual dysfunction', *British Medical Journal*, 341: c5050; Tiefer, L. (2010) 'Beyond the medical model of women's sexual problems: a campaign to resist the promotion of "female sexual dysfunction"', *Sexual and Relationship Therapy*, 25(2): 197–205.

Is medicalization a good or a bad thing? This question is not easily answered. Campaigns have been waged both for and against medicalization in particular circumstances. For example, it was a breakthrough for parents of children who died suddenly with no apparent cause when the medical profession agreed the new disease category Sudden Infant Death Syndrome (SIDS) (Byard and Krous, 2003). Growing acceptance of the diagnosis of dyslexia and recognition of the physiological basis of learning disabilities has been widely seen as a positive development, providing sufferers with support in place of stigma (read more about this subject in Chapter 9). On the other hand, there have been some 'diseases' which have been 'demedicalized'. In 1974, for example, the removal of 'homosexuality' from the *Diagnostic and Statistical Manual of Mental Disorders*, represented a step forwards for gay activists who challenged the idea that wanting to have sex with someone of your own gender should be seen as a symptom of some underlying biological abnormality (Conrad and Angell, 2004) (read more about the medicalization of sexuality in Chapter 7).

Medicalization enters into other areas of life as well. Zola highlighted the increasing role of health care professionals in the specialisms of psychiatry and public health. Psychiatry is involved in the management and control of social pathology, making decisions and influencing ideas about who may be deemed 'mad' or 'bad' (Szasz, 2007). For example, the 21-year sentence imposed on Anton Breivik for the murder of 77 people in Norway in 2011, hinged on complicated psychiatric evidence judged by the court to indicate that Breivik was sane at the time of the killings. Moral judgements are also involved in public health decisions, where the management and control of social environments involves making implicit judgements about what constitutes healthy and good neighbourhoods, parenting and personal behaviour (Zola, 1972).

Surveillance, Discourse and the Medical Gaze

In all societies, human beings have shared health-related norms and values: ideas about which foods are best to eat, what sexual behaviour is safe, when to wean children and how to relieve pain. In most societies, decisions about these issues have been essentially private. Modern societies are unique in having national institutions like the education, criminal justice and health care systems which aim, amongst other things, to transmit social norms and values. Prisons, schools and hospitals can be seen as institutions associated with efforts to monitor and improve our behaviour, a process referred to by the French sociologist Michel Foucault as **surveillance** (Foucault, 1977; Peterson and Bunton, 1997).

Surveillance: the monitoring and shaping of public behaviour.

An example of the subtle way surveillance works is the influence of Body Mass Index (BMI), a measure of body weight introduced in 1972. It has been suggested that almost a quarter of adults in England are obese, obesity being defined as having a BMI which is $30kg/m^2$ or more. Forty years ago, estimates of the extent of obesity suggested it was not such a problem as it is today. The change is not just because people are becoming more overweight. The adoption of the BMI measure changed what obesity means, who is obese and how common the problem is (Kennedy and Kennedy, 2010: 118).

It could be said that the idea of BMI has become part of social **discourse** about weight. For example, in many societies, people who see things that others cannot see have been viewed either as people with a special relationship with God or as being insane. Today, these experiences are referred to as hallucinations and they are explained in medical terms as resulting from taking particular drugs or a psychiatric disorder such as schizophrenia. This way of talking about having visions can be described as a modern discourse which makes sense of this experience in a particular way.

> Discourse: a way of talking about and thinking about something that influences the way we experience it.

There is one final concept that is relevant to this discussion. The way that a medical expert understands a person's body both reflects but also communicates medical discourse. Foucault called this the **medical gaze**. For Foucault, the medical gaze was an example of how social power works. Foucault's understanding of power is that it is not imposed from the top down, but works through society as if through a network of capillaries. Medical discourse does not only exist in the world of health care. Lay people participate in the transmission and repetition of influential discourses about health, not only in the way that we think and speak about health but in our routines and our habits. Every day we keep medical discourses alive when we brush our teeth after meals, wash our hands after using the toilet, choose one food over another or decide not to do something judged 'unhealthy'. Even when we behave in 'unhealthy' ways, we often know that we have 'erred'.

> Medical gaze: refers to the way in which medical professionals offer a view and a vision of how the human body works which comes to be adopted by lay people.

Risk

Finally, in our society, the issue of surveillance has also become tied up with the problem of risk. Nations, organizations and individuals have become increasingly concerned to establish what degree of risk they face and what they can do to minimize negative outcomes, whether economic, environmental or medical (Beck, 1992). In the field of public health, one obvious growth area related to risk is screening programmes, used to try to identify disease at an earlier and earlier stage. For example, we can identify individuals who have high blood pressure and are at risk of stroke. These efforts to 'head off' disease by making lifestyle changes before the disease can develop have changed the boundaries of abnormality. Individuals who might once have been judged healthy may now be identified as 'pre-symptomatic'. One result of this is the rise of a new category of patients who have been described as the 'worried well' (Royal Society of Public Health, 2005). They are not ill and intend to ensure it stays that way.

....

The New Genetics and the Worried Well

In recent years a wide variety of genetic tests have begun to be marketed to be bought directly by consumers online. Consumers send saliva to companies who then issue them with a report which gives their genetic susceptibility to diseases such as cancer, cardiovascular disease and diabetes. Genetic testing is marketed as offering consumers 'a new level of personalized medicine' (Navigenics.com). Some medical experts have advised caution, however. Whether a genetic predisposition results in the development of an illness depends on environmental factors: most of the variants covered by these tests 'are of extremely low predictive value' (Caulfield et al., 2010: 102). Focusing on the genetic factors may introduce a fatalism about illness. As Graham Watt argues, it was the removal of physical, social and economic hazards to health which resulted in the most significant advances in public health and longevity, not genetics (186). Genetic explanations for disease are also popular with the **eugenics movement**, who have historic links with fascism, and see discouraging or preventing some groups of people from having children as the route to a more robust society. Within the public health system, it is feared that allocation of resources for establishing risk for healthy people may be at the expense of those already unwell, and might even ensure a focus on the worried rich rather than the actually unhealthy poor.

Sources: Caulfield, T. et al. (2010) 'Direct-to-consumer genetic testing: good, bad or benign? *Clinical Genetics,* 77: 101–05; Watt, G. (2004) 'What will the new genetic information do for us?' *Journal of Health Services Research and Policy,* 9(3): 186–8.

....

CASE STUDY

Health Care: Power and Powerlessness

This chapter has explored some of the ways in which health care relates to the issue of social power. It considered some of the ways the issue of power is relevant to understanding health. This leaves a question which is not easy to answer: are medicine and the health care professions becoming more powerful? And where do lay people now stand in relation to medicine and power?

Illich suggested that the health care system has robbed us of the capacity for self-diagnosis. Traditional ways of understanding and looking after our bodies, handed down over centuries, were lost with the arrival of biomedicine, which Illich felt had left us vulnerable. However, the increasing role of lay people in health care (discussed in Chapter 1) and the growing use of the internet by people to educate themselves about their own health seem to suggest that there are now new opportunities for people to control their own wellbeing in relation to medicine (Ziebland and Wyke, 2012). Many aspects of public health today are reliant on lay involvement: managing chronic illness, health promotion and self-examination, for example. Some patients have educated themselves to the point of being experts in their own conditions and can be seen as auxiliaries in health care, hence the focus on 'patient-centred medicine' (Nettleton, 2004).

The rise of complementary medicine shows how lay people, as individual consumers, have been proactive about seeking alternatives to mainstream medicine. As members of patients' rights groups and self-help groups, lay people have demanded medical attention and research. Finally, a more negative example of our active role in our own care has been the rise of litigation against medical professionals. All of these developments suggest that, rather than becoming greater or lesser, medical power is instead becoming more dispersed. It is less concentrated in the hands of particular groups and more spread across society (Hughes, 2000; Gabe et al., 1994).

The picture is complicated, however. There are good reasons to question whether lay people are becoming more powerful. Globally, human health is increasingly threatened by inequality, war, recession and deregulation (more about this in Chapter 10). Power does not seem to be dispersed in low income countries where pharmaceutical companies have fought against the introduction of generic drugs for HIV/AIDS sufferers and use the majority world to test drugs that cannot legally be tested in developed countries (Cottingham and Berer, 2011). Though internet access is increasing all the time, not everyone can 'google' their own health problem, with only 30% of the world's population having access in 2012 (ITU, 2012). The internet also brings the potential for new health dangers. The ability to self-diagnose and self-prescribe via e-pharmacies, for example, means greater availability of unregulated and possibly dangerous products. A person's 'health literacy', their capacity to make use of information to enhance their health, also depends on the **social determinants of health,** structural factors such as social class, income and education (Chinn, 2011). Chapter 3 considers the crucial factor of social class.

> Social determinants of health: the circumstances in which people live, including the health system available to them.

Implications for Practice

The relationship between a health care professional and a service user is not just a relationship between two individuals, but has an important social aspect. Health care professionals can be seen as having a particular social role. Access to expertise arguably puts a health care professional in a position of power. The relationship between health care professional and service user is a relationship in which the professional is in a special position to communicate norms and values not only about healthy behaviour but about whether an issue should even be seen as a 'medical' issue and about what is accepted as normal in society. The rise of lay involvement in health care, however, means that service users, far from being passive in this relationship, are increasingly likely to use their own expertise to actively involve themselves in how their condition is understood and treated.

Summary

- Power involves the capacity of individuals and groups to influence others
- Health care is intimately involved with questions of social power, both reflecting and shaping them
- Lay people are not powerless but actively shape understanding and experience of health and illness

Exercise

Consider the following cases. Are these medical problems? What powerful individuals, groups or forces have influence on how each of these individuals understands their situation?

1. Daniel went to his GP feeling tired four months after the death of his father, was diagnosed as moderately depressed and offered anti-depression drugs.
2. Kirsty is convinced that only breast enhancement surgery will turn her life around.
3. Alastair has lung cancer which will eventually kill him, and he is refusing radiation therapy.

Further Reading

Armstrong, D. (1995) 'The rise of surveillance medicine', *Sociology of Health and Illness*, 17: 393–404.

Conrad, P. (2007) *The Medicalization of Society: On the Transformation of Human Conditions into Treatable Disorders*. Baltimore: John Hopkins University Press.

Lupton, D. (2012) *Medicine as Culture: Illness, Disease and the Body*. Third edition. London: Sage.

 Online readings

To access further resources related to this chapter, visit the companion website at www.sagepub.co.uk/russell

Nettleton, S. (2004) 'The emergence of e-scaped medicine', *Sociology* 38(4): 661–79.

3

Class

Key issues

- Our society is characterized by **class** inequalities, with different classes having unequal access to wealth, **power** and status
- People who are disadvantaged because of their class position also face major disadvantages in relation to their health
- These disadvantages can be understood as relating to material and cultural resources and **psychosocial factors**

Introduction

Most people have an idea what it means to say that someone is 'middle class' or 'working class'. Yet different people mean different things when they use these terms. This may be one reason why most of us don't feel very comfortable using these terms, whether we're discussing class in relation to ourselves or someone else. Just the idea of 'upper' and 'lower' class seems to suggest that some people are better than other people. The issue of social power, explored in Chapter 2, is closely related to the issue of **social class**. Social class is partly about how much power we have and our access to wealth and resources. Contrary to common belief, it is not very easy for most people to change the amount of wealth and power that they have in society, as this chapter will show. Social class has major implications for how long we will live, the good and bad health we experience across the course of our lives, and the cause of our death. This chapter will also explore reasons why class has this impact on our health.

> Social class: a grouping of people who share a similar situation in society based on their access to property and other resources.

A Short story of Class

A person's social class relates to issues such as their income and wealth (including possessions), their access to important resources, any power they might have over other people, and the amount of freedom they have to do what they want. Most societies have been unequal in all these regards, notably, in Ancient Greece, where many people were slaves. In medieval Europe, most people lived off the land but did not own their land and were under the power of landlords and the Church. The rise of science and **biomedicine**, described in Chapter 1, was associated with a new form of inequality, now known as **capitalism**. By the nineteenth century, landlords and the Church had moved aside for merchants and employers. Landless peasants became workers in workshops and factories, and later, in offices, producing a variety of goods that would be sold in the market for a profit. A society in which ownership of land was the most important basis for wealth and power became one where ownership of capital (that is, machinery, buildings, tools which could be used to create more wealth) became crucial.

In the mid-nineteenth century Karl Marx, a German philosopher who would become a leading figure in sociology, attempted to understand and challenge this new form of inequality in society. His close collaborator, Friedrich Engels, visited England and described the poverty and ill health he saw there at that time in a book called *The Condition of the English Working Class* (Engels, 1845/2006). Marx and Engels rejected the 'common sense' of the time, which viewed this poverty as the fault of the poor themselves. They drew attention to the importance of a person's relationship to the process of production in society – for example, whether they owned a factory or had to work in one – and how this economic reality seemed to set a person's fate in stone. Even the way that people choose to resist inequality, they argued, is constrained by their social position, with those who work for a living having no real means to improve their situation except by banding together as a group (Marx and Engels, 1848/2003).

For Marx and Engels, by banding together, members of the working class demonstrated the potential for an equal, classless society which could only be achieved by social revolution led from below. Despite their efforts, capitalism endured, but their ideas continue to be valuable as a basis for understanding inequality. In the early twentieth century, another German philosopher, Max Weber, suggested that class divisions were more complicated. He identified four main classes: the propertied class, white-collar workers, petty bourgeoisie (shopkeepers and small proprietors) and the working class. Weber also drew attention to other, more subjective factors that might influence a person's fate in society. For example, in addition to class, a person's **status** could make an important difference to their life chances. Political organization, or **party**, could also result in a better social position (Weber, 1976).

Status: honour or prestige acquired by different social groups in society that increases their social power.

Party: an organization which works to attain material advantages for its members and increase their social power.

Class Inequality in the Twenty-first Century

Since the nineteenth century, sociologists have noted many developments in the class structure of society. New types of occupations have arisen and others have declined, or even been lost forever. The kinds of resources that make a difference to a person's ability to improve their social position have changed over time; for example, knowledge and information have become much more important. There have been shifts in relationships between powerful groups in different parts of the world and in the degree to which **states** have attempted to control economic markets. Finally, the kinds of lifestyles associated with particular class groups in society are always evolving. There has been much discussion about these shifts and whether and in what ways they might have fundamentally changed the nature of inequality in society. What is mostly beyond debate amongst social scientists, however, is the continued existence of social inequality and the way that a person's social class constrains the kind of life they will have, how they are valued and the kind of choices they can make.

> The state/states: the government and national institutions they control that are paid for through taxation including the civil service, legal system, schools and universities.

Inequality between the richest and the poorest is greater, not less, than it was 150 years ago. The richest 1% of adults in the world own 40% of the planet's assets and the richest 10% account for 85% of the total while half of the world's adult population own barely 1% of global wealth (Davies et al., 2008: 7). Dramatically increased inequality has also been occurring in Britain. Figures from 2008, which probably underestimate the degree of inequality, show that between 1970 and 2005 the income of the top 0.1% of British society increased 694% while the income of the bottom 90% increased 48% (Wenchao et al., 2011). Today, the bottom 90% earn just 57.2% of all income (Dorling, 2012).

Measuring Class and Health

What does this inequality mean for human health? To answer this question, it is necessary to develop a way to compare people in terms of social class, and also to develop a way to compare the health of different people. The main approach taken today to measuring class is to group people by their occupation. There are two main scales that have been used. The first was the Registrar General's classification, shown in Table 3.1 as it appeared from 1921. For this scale, inspired by Weber's approach to class, occupations are organized into groups according to their 'general standing in the community' – in other words, the status of occupations.

Table 3.1 The Registrar General's Social Class classification

Class	Examples of occupations
I – professional	Lawyers, doctors
II – intermediate	Social workers, managers, shopkeepers
IIIa – skilled (non-manual)	Clerks, policemen, nurses
IIIb – skilled (manual)	Electricians, coal miners
IV – semi-skilled	Nursing assistants, farm workers, security guards
V – unskilled	Porters, cleaners

An updated version of this scale is still used today but it does have some limitations. For example, when the scale was devised, being a professional was a higher status job than it is today. There are many more professionals and managers in society today, but they do not all share similar status or life chances. There are also some important categories of people who do not even appear in this scale, for example, entrepreneurs, sporting stars, the unemployed and women working in the home.

Table 3.2 The National Statistics Socio-economic Classification system (NE-SEC)

Class	Examples of occupations
1 – higher managerial and professional	Doctors, lawyers, dentists, professors, professional engineers
2 – lower managerial and professional occupations	School teachers, nurses, journalists, actors, police sergeants
3 – intermediate	Airline cabin crew, secretaries, photographers, fire fighters, auxiliary nurses
4 – small employers and own account workers	Self-employed builders, hairdressers, fishermen, car dealers and shop owners
5 – lower supervisory and technical	Train drivers, employed craftsmen, foremen, supervisors
6 – semi-routine	Shop assistants, postal workers, security guards
7 – routine	Bus drivers, waiters and waitresses, cleaners, car park attendants, refuse collectors
8 – never worked or long-term unemployed	Students, people not classifiable, occupations not stated

From 2001 a new scale, the National Statistics' Socio-economic Classification system (NE-SEC) has been used (though the Registrar General's Scale does continue to be used also). The NE-SEC scale, shown in Table 3.2, was inspired by sociologists influenced by Marx, and defined class in a broader way, by taking in other criteria besides status. This scale takes into account factors such as whether the job is routine, whether it requires skills or qualifications and whether it gives someone power over others. The idea of '**socio-economic status**' recognizes the importance of both class and status to where we are each placed in the social hierarchy.

> Socio-economic status: a measure of social position which takes into account income, education and occupation.

The NE-SEC scale recognizes some subtle differences between occupations that became important over the course of the twentieth century. However, it is important to be aware that any way of measuring social class will have strengths and weaknesses. A scale that might be very useful for one purpose – say, comparing death rates across classes – may be less useful for a different purpose. Part of the work of social scientists involves deciding the best way to measure what you're studying. Comparing the health of different people is also not simple. How do you measure who is healthy and who is well?

Class and Mortality

One of the main ways the health of people has been measured is by looking at mortality rates – comparing the number of people from different social class backgrounds who have died within a certain time period. From looking at mortality rates we can see that people higher up the class scale live longer than those below. Figure 3.1, for example, demonstrates the difference that class made to the health of women aged 25 to 59 living in England and Wales in 2001 to 2008. The graph shows that more women from routine jobs died in this period than did women who worked as doctors and

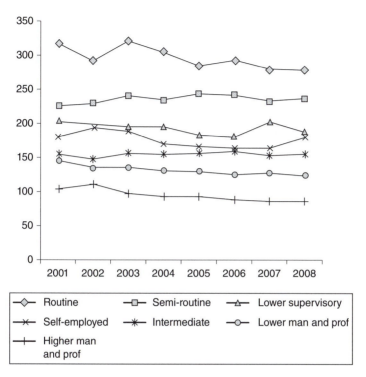

Figure 3.1 Age-standardised mortality rates by seven-class NS-SEC for 2001–08, women aged 25–59. England and Wales Rate per 100,000 person years

Source: Office for National Statistics

lawyers. Indeed, in general women from less well paid, lower status jobs were more likely to die.

Table 3.3 shows data collected about men in Scotland who died aged 20–59 between 1990 and 1992 (see Table 3.3). Though this survey is 20 years old, it illustrates well what is known as a 'social class gradient'. For this research, five basic social classes were identified, following the Registrar General's Scale. The table was created by sorting the numbers of men who died according to the cause of death. It shows a clear gradient associated with social class, with death rates for all conditions increasing from Class I to Class V. Statistics consistently show that mortality rates increase towards the bottom end of the social hierarchy. Moreover, the difference between the average age of death of men and women in Class V and those in Class I is getting wider. We are all living longer but the improvement has been faster for those in Class I (ONS, 2012a).

Table 3.3 Age standardised mortality (per 100,000 population) from selected causes within each social class group. Men aged 20–59, Scotland 1990–1992

Social class	Chronic lower respiratory diseases	Chronic liver disease	Accidents	Intentional self-harm and events of undetermined intent	Mental and behavioural disorders due to use of drugs	Mental and behavioural disorders due to use of alcohol	Assault
I	0	8	20	17	0	3	2
II	3	6	20	18	0	3	1
IIIa	7	15	20	24	0	6	2
IIIb	10	16	32	32	1	7	4
IV	13	12	34	35	0	6	4
V	25	33	82	80	5	26	21
-	3	3	19	29	2	5	3
All	8	12	29	30	1	6	4

Source: Leyland, Alastair H., Dundas, Ruth, McLoone, Philip and Boddy, F. Andrew (2007) Inequalities in Mortality in Scotland 1981–2001. Medical Research Council Social and Public Health Sciences Unit. Occasional Paper 16: 67 (Courtesy University of Glasgow)

Class and Morbidity

Comparing death rates is a useful and simple way to consider health differences across classes. Measuring ill health during life, however, is a little more complicated. There are two basic ways to do this. One is to use national surveys which ask people whether their health is good or poor. In Britain, the census and the General Household/Lifestyle Survey are two major surveys which have been used to gather this kind of information. Figure 3.2, for example, is based on the General Lifestyle Survey (ONS, 2011a) carried out by the Office of National Statistics. For this survey, people were asked to report whether they had a limiting long-standing illness or disability. It shows that, just as for mortality, social class makes a different to morbidity.

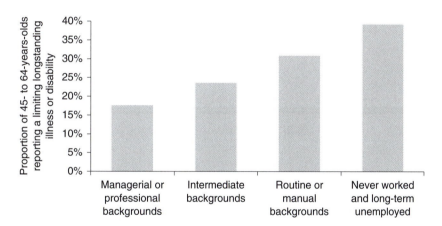

Figure 3.2 Adults aged 45–64 in routine and manual occupational groups are much more likely to have a limiting longstanding illness or disability than those from non-manual groups. The data is the average for the three years to 2009; Great Britain; updated Jan 2011

Source: General Lifestyle Survey, ONS. Available at: http://www.poverty.org.uk/61/index.shtml

Asking people about their health is a more subjective measure than counting the number of people who have died. However, over the years researchers have been able to check the **reliability** of this kind of measure by matching these self-assessments with other measures of health. For example, clinical surveys have been carried out to examine the extent of particular health problems such as angina or obesity. From comparing these different measures it has been found that rates of self-reported ill health are good predictors of a person's health status (Vaillant and Wolff, 2012). Research confirms that social class makes a difference to someone's likelihood of developing, for example, heart disease, cerebrovascular disease, asthma and diabetes. Figure 3.3 demonstrates this point in relation to ischaemic heart disease (heart disease associated with reduced blood supply to the heart) in Scotland. Other studies have shown that social class inequalities are reflected in birth weight, tooth decay and height in children. In turn, these conditions are implicated in other health problems developing. A low birth weight, for example, increases a person's chance of a number of health problems in later life (Spencer, 2008).

> Reliability: a finding is reliable when you can obtain the same result even when you use different ways of measuring the same thing.

A number of studies, the influential Black Report (1980), followed by the White-head Report (1987), the Acheson Report (1998) and the Marmot review (2010)

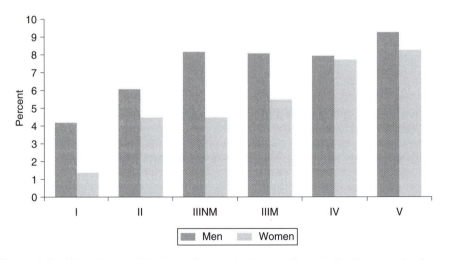

Figure 3.3   Prevalence of ischaemic heart disease (heart attack or angina) or stroke, by social class (Scotland, 1998)

Source: Scottish Health Survey 1998 Summary, available at: http://www.sehd.scot.nhs.uk/scottishhealthsurvey/sh8s-02.html

have all explored how class inequality continues to cause ill health. In relation to both mortality and morbidity the pattern is the same – the higher a person's position in the class hierarchy the better their health is likely to be (Dorling, 2013). However, as Figure 3.3 demonstrates, in addition to class differences in health patterns there are often also major differences between men and women. Gender is just one of a number of divisions in society which combine with class to make a difference to health patterns. Others include ethnicity, age and sexuality (and each of these divisions is the subject of a chapter in this book).

Poverty

Social class is connected to the problem of poverty. It is easy to see that for those on low incomes, lack of money can have many effects which lead to bad health, including stress, lack of money for healthy food and not being able to afford to heat your home when it is cold. To establish how many people in the UK are living in poverty, and establish what this means for their health, it is first necessary to define poverty.

One way to do this is to focus on people who do not have the bare minimum they will need just to stay alive. This is referred to as 'absolute poverty'. If a person's food intake is particularly inadequate their health will be impaired because of poor nutrition, reduced immunity and restricted growth. However, to describe poverty only in this strict way fails to capture changing lifestyles and the particular character of poverty in different societies. The bare necessities of life are not the same in every context. For this reason, researchers refer to 'relative poverty', poverty judged in relation to the normal standard of living in any given society (Townsend, 1979). In Britain, it is unusual for people to die from starvation, yet many die much younger than others because of disadvantage (Thomas et al., 2010). To identify those most in need, British social scientists use a measure of relative poverty (Rosenfeld, 2010). A line is drawn at 60% of median household disposable income (about £25,000 a year for a single household) and people in households whose income is below that line are considered to be living in poverty. People in this category will struggle to pay for food, heating, clothing, shoes and extras such as the occasional meal out or holiday (Cribb et al., 2012).

Research shows that people living in absolute or relative poverty are vulnerable to ill health throughout their lives. Today in Britain, 17–22% of the population (depending on whether housing costs are deducted) lives in relative poverty and around 13% live in absolute poverty. The UK has one of the highest rates of poverty in the industrialized world with almost one in three children (2.6 million) living in poverty, a percentage that is expected to rise (Cribb et al., 2012; Wenchao et al., 2011).

Factors Linking Class and Health

Much research carried out in Britain into health inequalities has shown that class disadvantage results in poorer health. In order to address the problem, it is important to understand why this happens. The 1980 Black Report investigated and rejected the idea that the ill health of the poor was a product of genetic inferiority. It showed that the conditions in which the poor were living were the reason for their ill health, not a product of it (Townsend et al., 1988). Some useful concepts for thinking about the reasons behind the relationship between poor health and class are cultural and material resources and psychosocial factors.

Cultural Resources

A common misconception about culture is to think of it as something that some people have more of than others. For instance, some people would see those who like different clothes or different music to themselves, as having more culture – or less. Another common idea of culture is that it is something associated with people from 'other' countries. However, all human beings share in culture. How we dress, what we eat for breakfast and how we present our Facebook page are all expressions of culture. Culture has a relationship with social class. People in more privileged social classes have more access to the kind of culture that demonstrates status in society and can be used to maintain or achieve access to wealth. **Cultural resources** might include formal skills learnt at school or university, or informal skills like knowing how to speak or behave in a way that will advantage you in a job interview. In general, the more cultural resources a person has, the more opportunities and choices are available to them in relation to employment, housing and lifestyle (Abel and Frohlich, 2012).

Other cultural resources include healthy habits built up from childhood, like eating fruit and vegetables every day, or knowledge about how to maintain mental health, for example, by taking 'time out' and seeking out friends when you are stressed. Research shows that there are some habits, beliefs and ways of doing things that are associated with ill health that are more common amongst people on low incomes. For example, many modern health problems are attributable to lifestyle factors, such as smoking, substance misuse (especially alcohol), lack of exercise and poor diet. Evidence suggests there is a strong class gradient in relation to smoking – the lower someone is on the social class scale, the more likely it is that they will smoke, and poorer people also tend to smoke more. People on a low income eat less fresh fruit and vegetables, fish and cheese, and more white bread, potatoes, sugar, lard and margarine. Poor diets associated with eating cheap processed foods are associated with bowel cancer. Poorer people also tend to exercise less (Stringhini et al., 2010).

Disadvantages faced by people on low incomes at school and at home also make it harder for them to acquire understanding and knowledge about how to live a healthy life compared with those higher up the class scale (Eichler et al., 2009). When improvements are made to health services, often it is those higher up the class scale who are able to make best use of them, what is known as the 'inverse care law' (Tudor Hart, 1971; DOH, 2009: 14). There is also evidence that people living in difficult economic circumstances are more likely to see poor health as a matter of luck or fate and therefore less likely to seek expert help (Ross and Mirowsky, 2013). For all these reasons, many measures to increase the 'cultural capital' of people disadvantaged by social class have been introduced in Britain in recent years. However, to understand the difference that cultural capital makes, it is necessary to see how cultural resources relate to material resources for people disadvantaged by social class.

> Cultural resources (or cultural capital): assets such as knowledge, skills and competencies that a person can use to improve their social position in society.

Material Resources

Michael Marmot, author of the influential Marmot review, argues that whilst access to health care and differences in lifestyle matter, the key determinants of health inequalities relate to the circumstances in which people are born and live throughout their lives (Marmot et al., 2010). These in turn arise from their different access to power and resources. Material resources, unlike cultural resources, are physical assets. They include all forms of economic capital, not only income and wealth but house, neighbourhood, furniture, clothing, personal and household items. In general, greater wealth means a greater chance of enjoying a better quality of housing, a safer neighbourhood, a shorter working week and more access to good food, nicer clothes, more comfortable transport, better schools and universities, private tuition, better holidays and an easy retirement.

Having more material resources means having more choices, such as being able to leave a job if it means having to work in an environment that is dangerous or toxic or being able to move to a different area to ensure children can go to a school where they feel safe. Having material resources makes it easier to acquire more material resources, whilst those who have few material resources are vulnerable to losing those they have. Low or semi-skilled work is much more likely to be dangerous work, which is part of the explanation for the much higher death rates from accidents shown for Class V illustrated in Table 3.3. For example, 5.3% of cancer deaths are caused by exposure to carcinogens at work (Health and Safety Executive, 2012). Poor housing often means damp housing, which is associated with asthma and low immunity (Suglia et al., 2010). Vitamin pills, disinfectant and toothpaste are some of the many health-related consumer items less available to those with less money.

As Chapter 5, 'Ageing', will discuss, studies which follow the lives of people over time (over their 'life course') have highlighted the importance of health in early life for later health. By the age of 50, people on low incomes are less likely to look after themselves to avoid ill health in the future. This is partly because they are already more unlikely to be unwell and to face stressful situations, with the result that the focus of their energy and resources are on dealing with present challenges (Ouwehand et al., 2009).

The issue of material resources is also key to understanding unhealthy beliefs, which endanger the health of those lower down the class scale. Poorer areas provide a more narrow range of food and transport costs prevent those on low incomes from going elsewhere to buy better food. For those on limited budgets cheap and filling food which will satisfy children for longer is an obvious choice. Exercising every day may be inevitable for someone employed in manual work but for those in less active occupations, working long hours and unable to afford child care, finding time to exercise may be very difficult. This is especially the case in neighbourhoods where there is a lack of green space and leisure facilities. Unhealthy habits like gambling, over-eating and smoking can only be understood in the context of these realities of life on a low income and the psychological challenges of coping in difficult circumstances (Stinghini, 2010) (see Case Study: Smoking on a Low Income).

CASE STUDY

Smoking on a Low Income

Researchers talked to single mothers living in poverty to try to understand why this group have high rates of smoking. Their study supports other research, which suggest that low-income women, whilst increasingly aware of the dangers of smoking, smoke as a way of coping with daily hassles and stress. Mothers living in conditions of material hardship often identified the time spent smoking cigarettes as the only time they had for themselves and cigarette smoking as the only activity they did for themselves. They described how they would turn to cigarettes when overwhelmed by too many demands, as a way of temporarily distancing themselves from their children, a strategy for managing their anger and protecting their children from it.

Source: Jun, Hee-Jin, Subramanian, S.V., Gortmaker, S. and Kawachi, I. (2004) 'Socio-economic disadvantage, parenting Responsibility, and women's smoking in the United States', *American Journal of Public Health*, 94(12): 2170–6.

Psychosocial Factors

In addition to material and cultural resources, one final factor is important in understanding the relationship between class disadvantage and ill health. Chapter 1 introduced the concept of 'psychosocial factors' when criticizing the biomedical model for reducing health issues to issues of biology. Psycho-social factors relate to aspects of life which are psychological but also social. They involve how a person's place in society impacts on their perceptions and experiences (Marmot and Wilkinson, 2009).

As discussed, being from a lower social class involves both cultural and material disadvantages. Research also suggests, however, that inequality itself has a striking effect on our health. Studies of civil servants have shown that there are health differences not only between one class and another but also between people higher and lower within the civil service hierarchy. These studies suggest that our awareness of our own place in society has a major impact on our health. Epidemiologists Richard Wilkinson and Kate Pickett present evidence that societies with a substantial gap between rich and poor are more vulnerable to ill health. More equal societies tend to be more healthy than those that are less equal. The explanation appears to be related to the psychological impact on a person of knowing that they are considered less valuable to others around them. Hierarchies cause stress for people who are lower in the pecking order, and this stress has a biological effect. Evidence suggests that sustained stress has a negative impact on the human immune system, making people more vulnerable to disease (Wilkinson and Pickett, 2010).

This research about psychosocial factors highlights that low social status can be damaging to our health. This is particularly important in the twenty-first century where disadvantaged groups are increasingly vulnerable to being shamed and stereotyped. In Britain, some political and media sources portray those on low incomes as 'scroungers' who are lazy, stupid or anti-social, unwilling to learn and who, by implication, deserve their disadvantaged circumstances (Skeggs, 2009; Tyler, 2008) (see Case Study: 'When you try to better yourself...'). Powerful groups in society are in a strong position to portray their own lifestyle and values as 'normal'. It can be said that they have 'symbolic capital' – the resources to ensure their vision of the world receives the most airplay (Bourdieu, 1991). An important aspect of challenging economic disadvantage in society involves rejecting images and talk that dehumanize people on low incomes (see Figure 3.4).

CASE STUDY

'When you try to better yourself they slap you back into place'

Rosemary Davidson and her co-researchers ran focus groups with people who knew one another living in different parts of Scotland and northern England, including deprived and more affluent areas. The researchers presented those in the groups with images and headlines about inequalities in health to see their reactions. Those from poorer areas easily understood the link between class and health and could give many examples from their own lives of how poor environments led to poor health, and of the link between a lack of material resources, stress and ill health. They told researchers how cramped conditions at home caused arguments or meant there was a lack of space for children to do homework. They told of how fear of street violence and frightening neighbours led to anxiety that fuelled ill health. It was also clear from the way they talked about these issues that they were angry about health inequalities and very aware and sensitive about being judged because of where and how they lived. By contrast, those from more affluent areas were more likely to reject the idea that disadvantage leads to poor health. These groups tended to explain the ill health of poor people in relation to factors such as a lack of education, criminal behaviour ('they're all shooting each other') taking illegal drugs, buying the wrong things and having the wrong priorities: '... *you'll still find that these poor people can afford their cigarettes'.*

Source: Davidson, R., Kitzinger, J. and Hunt, K. (2006) 'The wealthy get healthy, the poor get poorly? Lay perceptions of health inequalities', *Social Science and Medicine*, 62: 2171–82.

If stress caused by a sense of low worth and unhappiness is important to human health then one further resource that is important for people is **social capital**. Social capital involves networks and connections between people that foster trust, support and caring. Evidence shows that people who have more social capital tend to be healthier than those who do not. If someone has good social support, this can help them to maintain healthy behaviours in the face of stressors in their lives and a lower level of resources (Mulder et al., 2011).

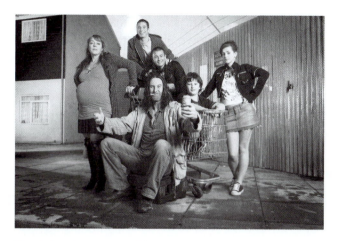

Figure 3.4 The television series *Shameless* represents one portrayal of working class life, but does it represent real life, stereotype or satire? Are these images empowering or are they demeaning?

Photograph courtesy Matt Squire

> Social capital: a resource that can be held by individuals which relates to their connectedness with others.

Social capital may also be related to one final factor related to class which has an important impact on health: place. Whilst people from all classes can be found in most areas, some areas have a higher proportion of people on low incomes and are much more prone to ill health. These places come to be unhealthy environments in which to live, due to a variety of factors including type of housing stock available, lack of recreational facilities, levels of vandalism and crime, pollution, poor local transport and amenities and lack of green space. Cultural factors such as lack of optimism and hope may also be involved, along with the quality of relationships between people (Shaw et al., 2005; Joshi et al., 2008).

Implications for Practice

Health care professionals undertake their work in a social class context. This means recognizing that the ability and willingness of people on low incomes to improve their own situation is constrained by the difficult circumstances in which they live, imposing particular personal challenges on them. In addition, as a health care professional your own place in the class structure of society will be important in relation to the opportunities available to you and pressures on you as you work with service users to support them to enhance their health.

Summary

- Social class has an enormous impact on human health
- Lack of access to material resources in crucial in the relationship between poor health and low social class
- Material disadvantage is linked to cultural disadvantage in complex ways

Exercise

1. List four 'bad habits' that might contribute to ill health for people on low incomes.
2. For each of the 'bad habits' identify two ways that a lack of material resources might cause problems which make that habit more likely amongst people on low incomes.

Further Reading

Bartley, M. (2004) *Health Inequality: An Introduction to Concepts, Theories and Methods*. Cambridge: Polity Press.

Dorling, D. (2013) *Unequal Health: The Scandal of Our Times*. Bristol: Policy Press.

Wilkinson, R. and Pickett, K. (2010) *The Spirit Level: Why More Equal Societies Almost Always Do Better*. Second edition. London: Allen Lane.

Online readings

To access further resources related to this chapter, visit the companion website at www.sagepub.co.uk/russell

Graham, H. (2012) 'Smoking, stigma and social class', *Journal of Social Policy* 41(1): 83–99.

4

Ethnicity

Key issues

- The idea that there are sub-species of human beings (races) is not suggested by the genetic evidence
- The different experiences of people from different ethnic backgrounds are mainly due to society rather than biology
- People from ethnic **minority groups** face particular disadvantages in relation to health

Introduction

Chapter 3 explored the implications of the sensitive issue of class for human health. The issue of **ethnicity** is perhaps even more sensitive. Some of us would prefer not to talk or even think about ethnic differences, but focus on what we have in common. However, the idea that humanity can be sub-divided into different racial groups has been influential in our society and is reflected, even today, in health patterns. Some people are likely to face disadvantages that affect their health in a negative way because of their ethnic background. This chapter seeks to clarify just how these patterns came about.

A Short History of Race

Most human societies have held some negative beliefs about people from other groups. People in Ancient Greece and Rome, for example, distrusted outsiders

(Gruen, 2011). The idea that some groups of people are *innately* inferior to others, however, is comparatively recent (Miles and Brown, 2003: 39). In the eighteenth century, the social changes we associate with **the Enlightenment** and the industrial revolution produced a new way of thinking about human difference. European countries had begun to portion out the globe in their search for greater power and wealth, making satellites of areas of the world which had previously hosted powerful civilizations, in Africa, the Middle East and Asia. Behind this colonial drive were ideas and values that reflected the rise of a new elite who championed science, rationality and success due to 'merit' against religious and hereditary elites. Yet much of the wealth of this group was acquired by the capture and sale of African people to plantations in the Caribbean and America. Though slavery was eventually abolished, white Europeans developed so-called 'racial science' to justify the treatment of African slaves and colonized peoples (Hall, 1996) (see Figure 4.1). A medical scientist, for example, developed the diagnosis drapetomania, a supposed disease characterized by an 'irrational' desire of slaves to run away from their masters (Jarvis, 2008). The image shows three skulls, one belonging to a white man, identified as 'Greek', the one beneath it belonging to a black man, described here as a 'negro', and the third at the bottom belonging to a chimpanzee. It illustrates the influence of Social Darwinism in the 19th century, whose followers attempted to use Darwin's theories of evolution as justification for a racial order in which African people were routinely treated as animals.

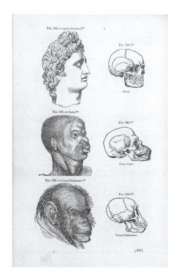

Figure 4.1 Image from J.C. Nott and George R. Gliddon (1854) *Types of Mankind*

By the early decades of the twentieth century, the idea that humans belonged to racial groups with distinct inherited characteristics was very influential. The **eugenics movement**, popular at that time, also identified as genetically inferior gay and disabled people, people with learning disabilities and mental illness, and the poor. In Nazi Germany, eugenics lay behind the systematic murder of millions of Jews, black people, disabled and gay people and other 'undesirables' considered to be a genetic danger to future generations (Bashford and Levine, 2010). It was not until the mid-twentieth century that belief in the idea of race was seriously challenged. The word '**racism**' was only first used as we understand it today in 1943 (Benedict, 1943). In the years following the Holocaust, struggles by people in the **majority world** for political independence together with the US civil rights movement further undermined the superiority of the Western world and challenged those who discriminated on the basis of race. Yet despite this shift, the idea of race remains influential, and continues to distort relationships between people. This way of thinking freezes people into categories, gives them fixed qualities and does not take into account the wider social circumstances in which relationships between different peoples are played out. The idea of racial difference also continues to haunt discussions about ethnicity and health.

> Eugenics movement: the 'science' of controlling human breeding to discourage the birth of people cast as genetically inferior, including disabled and gay people and those from ethnic minority groups.
>
> Racism: words or actions which reflect a view that human beings can be divided into sub-species, and that some sub-species are superior to others.

Race and Ethnicity

In our society it is 'common sense' to believe that people who look similar on the outside are similar on the inside too. In our minds we sort people into different races, and we do this almost automatically, in the same way we sort people into men and women, young and old. For sociologists, however, common sense ideas often reveal more about our society and dominant ways of thinking than they do about the way things really are. Some of the ways we routinely think about the world can be shown to be quite wrong. The idea of race is an excellent example.

In our society, skin colour in particular is often used to judge where a person's ancestors might be from. It is assumed that people who look alike came from the same 'gene pool' at some point in the past and that surface similarities indicate other, underlying similarities. It is assumed that human beings belong to separate groups – African, Asian, European, for example – that are genetically different to one another. However, recent genetic science shows that when the genes of many different people are compared, the patterns that are found do not fit with common sense ideas about race (Fortier, 2011; Malik, 2009; Carter, 2007). Due to migration over the centuries, many of us have ancestors from all over the world (Moffat and Wilson, 2011). If we consider any single characteristic that is passed down from one generation to the next, it is found that there are few, if any, characteristics that belong only to one ethnic group and not to others. Genetic research has highlighted that as a species, human beings are very genetically similar to one another. If we believe we see a 'typical' European or a 'typical' African when we meet someone, our minds are doing some creative work that we are not conscious of.

Another way to say this is to say that our ideas about race are socially constructed. This is a very important idea and will be discussed again in several other chapters in this book. As members of our society, we participate in the culture of our society and learn the habits, beliefs and values of its members. More than that, as members of society we learn to experience and understand the world in the way that others in our society understand it. This is what is meant by the idea of **social construction.**

Social construction: a concept used to emphasize the social or cultural rather than biological basis of social divisions and differences.

Ethnicity is a term that is used to talk about differences between human beings that emphasizes our cultural rather than biological connection with our family, community and forebears. Ethnicity is a way we identify who we are and how we are different to others. In particular, it involves thinking about ourselves as sharing a culture with other people, for example, a shared history, language and religion (Bloch and Solomos, 2009; Karner, 2007).

> Ethnicity: an identity that locates a person as belonging to a group who see themselves as distinct on the basis of shared characteristics such as kin, history, heritage, language, religion and nationality.

Ethnic Minority People in Britain – profile

When we talk about ethnic minorities in Britain, it is common for people to think about migration. However, it is worth bearing in mind that many migrants in Britain are from relatively wealthy white communities in countries such as Germany and South Africa (ONS, 2012b). In addition, most ethnic minority people in Britain today are not migrants, but the UK-born descendents of migrants – roughly half of the Indian, Pakistani, Bangladeshi, Black Caribbean and Black African people in Britain were born here (Ahmad and Bradby, 2009: 5). Inter-marriage also complicates the issue of ethnicity and the experience of recently arrived migrant workers from Central and Eastern Europe confirms that of Irish and Jewish migrants; being white does not necessarily protect people from ethnic discrimination and inequality (Spencer et al., 2007). What is clear from the evidence is that the 14% of the British population classified as being from an ethnic minority (ONS, 2012b) are more likely to live in poor housing, be unemployed or in low wage employment, live in poverty and been in trouble with the police (Bloch and Solomos, 2009).

> Ethnic minority: a group of people who have a shared language, culture and way of life that is different from the majority in the society where they live.

Since 1991, the British census has asked people about their ethnicity, enabling researchers to identify patterns of disadvantage for different ethnic groups. This has highlighted that different ethnic groups have different histories and so what is true for one group may not be true for another. Most Asian groups, for example, are well-established in Britain, with a large proportion of members having being born in Britain. Polish people, on the other hand, have mostly only recently arrived and their lives and health problems may reflect these differences. In addition, however, the idea of ethnic 'groups' has itself been criticized. People who identify themselves as having the same ethnicity may differ in relation to social class, gender, age, generation, sexuality, religion and whether they live in rural or urban areas. Ethnic 'groups' encompass many different lifestyles and individuals within them may have quite different ideas about what it means to be part of that ethnic 'group' (Brubaker, 2004).

Health Differences Related to Ethnicity

On the whole (with some exceptions) ethnic minority people have worse health than white people in Britain (Mathur et al., 2013: 9). One exception is that most ethnic minority people have lower rates of disease and mortality from respiratory problems, lung cancer and breast cancer (Nazroo, 2010). However, different groups also have different histories and different health profiles.

Perhaps the oldest ethnic minority group in Britain is the Irish. Irish people living in England and Wales have higher rates of morbidity (especially cardiovascular disease) and mortality, and are vulnerable to depression and suicide, patterns which persist in later generations (Sproston and Mindell, 2006; Das-Munshi et al., 2013). Apart from the Irish, several of the biggest ethnic minority groups in Britain mostly migrated in the years following 1948 when changes to the law were made with the aim of encouraging migration to fill labour shortages. These countries had previously been colonies of Britain, notably India and the new countries created following Indian independence, Pakistan and Bangladesh, as well as countries in the Caribbean.

People who identify themselves as Indian in Britain migrated or descended from those who migrated to Britain from the northern Indian state of Punjab or the western Indian state of Gujerat, with numbers peaking in the late 1960s. In terms of religion, they were mainly Hindus and some were Muslims. They settled in a number of different regions and industries. Today, the health levels of this group and their descendents are comparable to whites, though they have somewhat higher rates of diabetes, cardiovascular disease and depression (Garrett et al., 2012; Sproston and Mindell, 2006). Other Indians came to Britain through Africa, including those expelled from

Uganda in the 1960s. African Asians and East African Asians appear to have similar health profiles to Indian groups; that is, they are comparatively healthy. One other group, which also appear to be fairly healthy, despite problems of access to health services, is the Chinese (Green et al., 2006).

Other groups from Asia are, on average, not so healthy. Those who migrated here in the 1950s and 1960s from Pakistan were mostly land-owning farmers who came to work as semi-skilled labour but faced unemployment when industries like the textile industry declined. The people who arrived from Bangladesh in the late 1970s faced even worse circumstances. The conditions experienced by those in these groups are reflected in their health patterns. Pakistanis and Bangladeshis have rates of coronary heart disease (CHD) significantly higher than whites and both men and women from these groups are more likely to report bad or very bad health. Whilst Indian people are three times as likely as white people to suffer from diabetes, Pakistanis and Bangladeshis are five times as likely (Sproston and Mindell, 2006; Chaturvedi, 2003).

African Caribbeans were also encouraged to come to Britain in large numbers in the 1950s and 1960s, until a new law changed this in 1972. Many worked in public transport and the NHS, settling in big cities like London and Birmingham. They have some distinctive health patterns, for example, high rates of hypertension, stroke, and type 2 diabetes mellitus, but up to 50% lower mortality from CHD (Harding, 2004). This group also appears to have high rates of psychosis (see Case Study: African Caribbean Psychosis in Britain) yet low rates of suicide.

Black Africans, a separate group, first arrived in Britain in large numbers in the 1990s, fleeing conflict and political unrest in countries like Somalia and Zimbabwe, with the biggest groups from Nigeria and Ghana. Their economic circumstances tend to be relatively favourable and, like African Caribbeans, those from these groups have much lower rates of heart disease compared to the white population but significantly higher rates of hypertension, stroke and diabetes (Chaturvedi, 2003; Tillin et al., 2006).

There are other groups whose health we know little about. The country from which the second-largest number of foreign-born residents come, after India, is now Poland (ONS, 2012b). Smaller numbers of people from other parts of Central and Eastern Europe, mostly younger, mainly single people coming for work, migrated to Britain from 2004 onwards (Trevena, 2009). Central and Eastern Europeans have faced overcrowding in rented accommodation, discrimination in housing and harassment, with alarming levels of poverty, depression and suicide being reported amongst Polish migrants (Lakasing and Mirza, 2009; Rolfe and Metcalf, 2009; Shields, 2008).

Finally, asylum seekers in Britain are a small group from many different countries who make up just 0.3% of the British population. They are labelled as 'asylum seekers' because they have applied for asylum after losing their homeland, and are only allowed to be described as 'refugees' when they are granted the right to live in the UK. Both groups have health problems which reflect their extreme poverty and vulnerability in British society (Jayaweera, 2010).

These profiles give some idea of ethnic health patterns. However, there are several reasons to be cautious about the picture painted here. When researchers first began to look seriously at ethnic minority health patterns they assumed Indian, Pakistani and Bangladeshi people (South Asians) would have fairly similar health patterns. We now know these groups have quite different patterns. Even within those groups, divisions are apparent. People born in India, for example, come from different regions and have different religions. Grouping them all together under the category 'Indian' may mean that these differences are hidden. In addition, the more we learn about the health of ethnic minority people, the more we see the importance of other social divisions. Men and women in the same ethnic group, for example, may have quite different patterns of health reflecting their different roles. Different generations also have different patterns of health (Garrett et al., 2012).

Explanations

How are we to explain these health patterns associated with ethnicity? The first British people interested in ethnic minority health were researchers concerned to protect the white population from exotic diseases that might be brought in by foreigners. Ethnic minority health was understood through a racist lens that framed 'Western' lifestyles, culture and science as superior. Even today, explanations for ethnic health patterns continue to reflect outdated ideas about what ethnicity means and what makes ethnic minority people different to the majority.

Genetic Differences

Some human health conditions are related to inherited genetic differences. One example is sickle cell disorders, painful diseases which result when two carriers of a particular genetic irregularity have children together. Another is Tay-Sachs disease, caused by a genetic mutation which is more common amongst some populations than others. These are just two examples of diseases which are statistically more likely to occur within particular populations. Other examples include diabetes and cardiovascular disease (Mathur et al., 2013). Does this mean, however, that those diseases are 'racial'?

The example of sickle cell disorders is useful for demonstrating how the idea of race can distort our understanding of health differences in unhelpful ways. The genetic irregularity associated with sickle cell disease occurs in areas of world where malaria has been common. The irregularity protects people from malaria. In West Africa, one in four people can carry these genes and carriers can also be found amongst Cypriots, Pakistanis and the Chinese. Knowing about the genetic basis of this disease is very important for prediction and diagnosis. However, in Britain, the first cases of sickle cell disease were mostly amongst Africans and African Caribbeans. Racial thinking led to the assumption that sickle cell disease was a 'Black disease', even though many African people are not at risk for these diseases and many carriers are not African. The misconception that sickle cell disorders are 'Black diseases' could even lead to fatal misdiagnoses (Dyson and Atkin, 2011; Witzig, 1996).

This example highlights the dangers of assuming that all people who identify themselves as being of the same ethnicity are more genetically similar to one another than to others. Indeed, the idea of race has been identified by leading geneticists as an obstacle to helpful research about ethnic minority health. Yet racial explanations for disease remain popular. For example, the idea that genetics must lie behind higher rates of hypertension suffered by Africans in many countries has been popular, even though careful research suggests these rates are associated with the conditions of poverty and poor eating experienced by Africans in many places where they live (McKeigue, 2001). In recent years, some doctors have made the mistake of assuming that certain health problems in South Asian children are the result of marriage between cousins, even where the parents in question are not cousins or the illness is unlikely to be related to cousin marriage (Ahmad and Bradby, 2009: 7).

Cultural Differences

Other popular explanations for ethnic minority health patterns focus on cultural habits presumed shared by those in the group. Despite their popularity, only one of these habits, smoking, follows a clear 'ethnic' pattern. Smoking is the largest preventable cause of death in Britain and is largely a habit of the poorest and most disadvantaged socio-economic groups. As ethnic minority people are more likely to be poor and disadvantaged, you might expect higher rates of smoking amongst ethnic minority people. However, the picture is more complicated. For example, women in most ethnic groups smoke less than men, for a cultural reason common across ethnic groups: smoking has tended to be viewed as unfeminine (Nazroo, 2010).

In addition, different attitudes associated with religion have an impact on smoking patterns. The Sikh religion, for example, frowns on smoking, and Indian Sikhs, as well as Hindus, have low smoking rates resulting in lower rates of heart disease. Whilst Islam does not discourage smoking, Muslims are more likely than Christians to give religious or cultural reasons (such as not wanting to disrespect parents) for not smoking, and Pakistanis, who are mostly Muslim, have low rates of smoking and low rates of respiratory illness and lung cancer (Sproston and Mindell, 2006; Millward and Karlsen, 2011). Religion may also play some role in the higher rates of abstinence and lower levels of drinking of Asian and African Muslims whose religion has strictures against drinking. Some other groups, such as the Irish and first-generation Sikh men, drink more than average, with consequent health effects such as higher rates of liver cirrhosis (Hurcombe et al., 2010).

Another health-related lifestyle factor which has received much attention is diet. Like smoking, a poor diet is a risk factor for CHD. Certain habits, such as cooking with ghee, have been linked with higher rates of heart disease and diabetes. However, not all South Asians traditionally use ghee in cooking, and many South Asians have begun to use oil instead or have cut down their fat consumption in other ways. In addition, young people from South Asia, especially those busy with work or study, are more likely to eat a combination of home-cooked food and relatively unhealthy 'fast food' (Lucas et al., 2013).

The issue of 'fast food' highlights the difficulty of trying to match unhealthy eating with ethnicity. Unhealthy habits and beliefs are common in all ethnicities in Britain. Darr et al. (2008), for example, surveyed white and ethnic minority patients with heart disease and found that many shared a strong belief that fate was an important factor in their contracting the disease. Cultural habits that effect health are also related to the circumstances in which we live. For example, South Asian women seeking to improve their health have spoken of the difficulty of finding safe places to walk alone for exercise in city areas. Sporting centres and other bodies can exclude Muslim women by failing to facilitate access to gender segregated activities that cater to their sensitivities (Long et al., 2009) (see Figure 4.2).

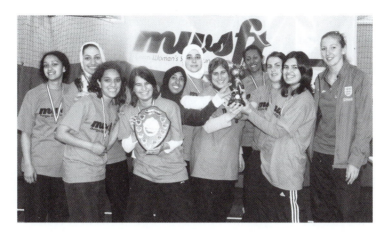

Figure 4.2 Muslim Women's Sport Foundation Cobras, winners of the 2010 Futsal Festival, Kilburn

Photograph courtesy Muslim Women's Sport Foundation

The focus on genes and culture to explain ethnic minority health patterns reveals that we live in a society in which the idea of racial difference continues to be used as a way to understand differences which are better understood in other ways. James Nazroo, a leading expert on ethnicity and health in Britain, commented that these kinds of explanations persist despite more than 100 years of research exposing their limitations (Nazroo, 2010: 118). The problem with focusing on genetic or cultural differences is that this tends to make ethnic differences more important than they really are. Ethnic identity is a product of society. It is defined in living relationships between people which are complex and always changing.

Migration

One factor that does have a clear impact on ethnic minority health is migration. People who have migrated have lived their life in two or more countries. Therefore, it is to be expected that their health will reflect the lives they lived and the pressures they were under in those other countries, not only the country in which they currently live. Contrary to media portrayals of migrants bringing disease to our shores, it would be more accurate to say that it is living in Britain that brings ill health to migrants. Those who decide to take the risk of moving to another country tend, on average, to be healthier than those left behind. For certain infections, including tuberculosis (TB), HIV and malaria, migrants are more likely to be sufferers than non-migrants, but the rate of these infections amongst migrants is very low, as is the chance of infecting others through normal contact (Health Protection Agency, 2006; Wagner et al., 2013). However, the comparative healthiness of migrants when they arrive in Britain decreases over time (Jayaweera, 2010: 3).

One explanation for this is that the migration process is stressful and disruptive (Mathur et al., 2013). However, this cannot be the only explanation, since this higher risk of ill health is also shared by the children and grandchildren of migrants. Those of us who are second and third generation have not experienced the stress of migration. As Figure 4.3 shows, for example, rates of diabetes amongst people of West African descent are clearly related to the countries where they live. Some other factors besides migration itself must therefore be involved (Health Protection Agency, 2006).

Socio-economic Factors

In the previous chapter, it was argued that the less wealth, power and status you have, the more likely it is that you will also have poor health. The patterns of health problems seen amongst ethnic minority people make more

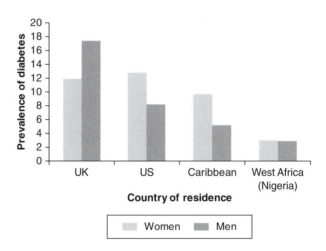

Figure 4.3   Prevalence of diabetes by mean BMI and sex in populations of West African origin: the ICSHIB Study, 1996

Source: Cooper R., Rotimi C., Kaufman J.S., et al. (1997) 'Prevalence of NIDDM among populations of the African diaspora', *Diabetes Care*, 20(3): 345. Available at http://care.diabetesjournals.org/content/20/3/343.full.pdf

sense if we look at the class profiles of different ethnic groups. For example, the personal wealth of someone from a Bangladeshi background in Britain is on average less than that of someone from India. Given what we know about the impact of social class on health, you would expect that Bangladeshi health would tend to be worse on average than Indian health. This is exactly what the statistics suggest (Ahmad and Bradby, 2009). Indeed, it is likely that **socio-economic** factors may explain most ethnic minority health patterns, though these factors have not been easy to identify (Nazroo, 2010). These socio-economic disadvantages are then translated into lower birth weights for ethnic minority children, which in turn have an impact on the health of those children when they grow up (Davey Smith, 2000).

Other factors may also have an impact on class which are not related to ethnicity as such, but are socio-economic 'side effects' of coming from another country. For example, language barriers are one important factor affecting the living standards of ethnic minority people who are migrants from countries where English is not their first language. Other factors that systematically affect the statistics for particular groups do not appear to be related to either ethnicity or migrant status. For example, it has been suggested that African Caribbeans are more likely to live in single adult households, which may have increased their vulnerability to disadvantage (Sharpley et al., 2001). 'Ethnicity' does not explain every aspect of the lives of white people. Likewise, there is no reason to assume it can explain every aspect of the lives of ethnic minority people.

Racism

Regardless of the many differences within and across ethnic groups, there is one thing that ethnic minority people have in common: a history of discrimination. This unequal treatment is reflected in patterns of disadvantage in relation to housing, employment, criminal justice, education and healthcare. Institutions like the NHS, the police force, schools, the courts, housing and employment agencies and welfare departments also bear this history in ways of doing things which, whilst they may not be deliberately racist, nonetheless result in worse service for ethnic minority people.

This problem of **institutional racism** was first officially admitted by the police force following the 1999 inquiry into the failure of the police to bring to justice the murderers of teenager Stephen Lawrence in 1993 (McLaughlin, 2009). Equality legislation in the twenty-first century – especially the **Equality Act 2010** – has aimed to redress institutional racism but much evidence attests to the failure to ensure equal opportunities for ethnic minority people in many contexts. One example that is particularly notable is how the operation of criminal justice and mental health services works to perpetuate an over-representation of African and African Caribbean youth in the courts, in prison and on medication for psychosis (see Case Study).

Institutional racism: where an institution discriminates against ethnic minority people because of ingrained attitudes and practices that work to disadvantage ethnic minority people.

Equality Act 2010: legislation designed to protect people in Britain from discrimination on the basis of age, disability, gender assignment, marriage and civil partnership, pregnancy and maternity, race, religion or belief, sex or sexual orientation.

CASE STUDY

African Caribbean Psychosis in Britain

African Caribbean people in Britain have a very high risk of being diagnosed with **psychosis**. Rates of psychosis of African Caribbean people living in Caribbean countries are similar to those of white people in Britain, so genetics cannot be the reason. It is known that people who migrate from the majority world to countries where most people are white have an increased risk of schizophrenia. However, migration alone cannot explain the problem either, since the children of African Caribbean migrants, born in Britain, are also at a markedly higher risk. One factor that has been much discussed is institutional racism. African Caribbeans are more likely than white people to be admitted to hospital compulsorily and twice as likely to have experienced involuntary admission. They are significantly more likely than other ethnic groups to have experienced police contact including police referrals into hospital and imprisonment. In a situation where a psychiatrist is faced with a person who is agitated and perhaps frightened, it has been suggested that a diagnosis of psychosis may permit the psychiatrist to restrict the liberty of someone they may find threatening. Yet evidence also suggests that there are pressures on African Caribbean people which do 'break' some individuals. Recent research has highlighted a powerful link between trauma and psychosis and African Caribbean people are more likely to experience social adversity in the form of unemployment, poor housing, childhood abuse or disrupted family life, social isolation, problems associated with city living and experiences of victimisation and discrimination. You can read more about the role of childhood adversity on mental health in Chapter 9.

Sources: Fernando, S. (2010) 'DSM-5 and the "Psychosis risk syndrome"', *Psychosis: Psychological, Social and Integrative Approaches,* 2(3): 196–8; Luhrmann, T.M. (2010) 'The protest psychosis: how schizophrenia became a black disease' (review article), *Am J Psychiatry,* 167: 479–80.

Psychosis/psychotic disorders: disorders whose main symptom is impairment of a person's ability to perceive reality, expressed mainly in delusions or hallucinations.

Institutional racism affects the health of ethnic minority people in a number of ways. For example, discrimination by housing agencies results in ethnic minority people living in worse quality housing so they are more likely to live in damp unhealthy conditions. Discrimination in the labour market, particularly in the context of recession, results in higher rates of unemployment and lower wages, which also has an impact on health (Bloch and Solomos, 2009). To the extent that institutions like the NHS also fail to provide equal treatment, ethnic minority people may be discouraged from engaging with the health service, to their detriment (Bécares and Das-Munshi, 2013).

In addition, there is one way in which racism in society has a simple, direct and potentially devastating impact on the health of ethnic minority people. A growing body of evidence testifies to the psychosocial health consequences of stress caused directly by racial harassment and violence and indirectly through experiences of discrimination and 'status'-related hurt. A survey of Muslims following the events of 9/11, for example, shows experiences of direct and indirect discrimination increased after that time and suggests links between mental health problems in this group and reports of being abused in relation to those events (Sheridan, 2006).

The limited evidence that exists about the health of asylum seekers suggests that hostility from wider society contributes to their already highly vulnerable mental and physical health (O'Donnell et al., 2007). Roma and Irish traveller communities are also particularly vulnerable in this regard (Van Hout and Staniewicz, 2012). These kinds of factors may partly explain why the difference between ethnic minority and white health becomes greater as people age. In youth, racial discrimination may not be sufficient to affect someone's health, but over time, the effects accumulate and the body feels the cost, a process that has been described as 'weathering' (Nazroo, 2010).

Health Benefits of Ethnicity?

Despite this negative picture, other research explores how ethnic minority people have adapted their lives to cope with the stresses and disadvantages of life in a racist society. These adaptations may have health benefits. For example, neighbourhoods with a high proportion of ethnic minority people may benefit from social capital built up because of the need to support one another in an, at times, unfriendly society (Bécares, 2009; Stafford et al., 2010). Ethnic groups may offer a source of identity and connection which is good for people's health.

In summary, ethnic minority health patterns reflect the continued influence of racial thinking and institutional racism in our society. However, as individuals we interpret our own **identity** in the context of our past and our family's past. Our ethnicity is one part of who we are, but what our ethnicity means for how we eat, dress and live our lives is complicated. No ethnic group has fixed habits or customs which are the same for everyone in the group. To live a healthy life each of us modifies and adapts values and ways of doing things which we inherited from our parents and grandparents (see Case Study: Attitudes Towards Termination of Pregnancy...). Disadvantage is an undeniable part of the story of ethnic minorities in Britain but so are creativity, flexibility and resilience.

Identity: how we categorize ourselves in relation to others.

CASE STUDY

Religious Attitudes Towards Termination of Pregnancy in Cases of Inherited Haemoglobin Disorder

Researchers in England spoke to people identified as being at risk of haemoglobin disorders, associated with symptoms such as chronic acute pain, severe bacterial infections and tissue death. They asked Pakistani Muslims, Indian Sikhs and Hindus and African Caribbean Christians how they would approach the decision of whether to terminate a pregnancy if testing revealed the child would have a haemoglobin disorder. Their answers highlight the similarities between different religious groups, rather than their differences. Participants tended to agree that whilst they would take into account the position of their religion on the issue of termination, it is essentially a private decision. Religion was not seen as offering fixed rules about moral decisions. Whilst taking a life might be regarded as a sin, this was balanced against the moral value of preventing suffering. Whilst some Pakistani Muslims stressed the importance of early screening, following some Islamic guidance on the issue, they also emphasized: 'It's not a robot religion, it depends on the situation'. All felt that the severity of the condition is as important, if not more important, as religious beliefs. Hindus, Sikhs and Muslims generally agreed that because the disorder thalassaemia, in particular, meant 'a lifetime of suffering', termination was justified. As one Muslim man said: '(r)eligion wouldn't come into it really. It would be my own ethics. I wouldn't want to put a child through all that pain and suffering'. The men who participated also agreed that as the one who must carry the child, it is the pregnant woman who must make the final decision.

Source: Atkin, K., Ahmed, S., Hewison, J. and Green, J.M. (2008) 'Decision-making and ante-natal screening for sickle cell and thalassaemia disorders: to what extent do faith and religious identity mediate choice?' *Current Sociology*, 56(1): 77–98.

•••

Implications for Practice

What does this mean for health professionals? NHS policy recognizes that to ensure equality staff should be flexible and recognize that different people have different needs. One way to show recognition of the need for racial equality in health care has been to provide relevant information about religious and cultural characteristics of different groups for professionals. In addition, ethnic minority people themselves must be at the heart both of managing their own health and of delivering service improvements.

Summary

- Racial thinking and practices that discriminate against ethnic minority people continue to be a feature of our society
- The factors resulting in overall worse health for ethnic minority people are complex, but socio-economic factors are most important
- The meaning of ethnicity is not fixed or stable

Exercise

'I think it's a shame when a culture can't see that something they're doing which is near and dear to their wishes is causing such havoc among their children.' (Cited in Ahmad et al., 2000: 39–40)

This is a quote from a white health care practitioner, making a mistaken connection between rates of congenital deafness and the common South Asian practice of marriage between cousins. Can you think of other examples of 'culture blaming'? Why do you think health care practitioners engage in 'culture blaming'? What would be a better way to understand a health pattern which appears to be associated with ethnicity?

Source: Ahmad, W.I.U. et al. (2000) 'Causing havoc to their children': parental and professional perspectives on consanguinity and childhood disability', in W.I.U. Ahmad (ed.) *Ethnicity, Disability and Chronic Illness*. Buckingham: Open University Press, 28–44.

Further Reading

A useful starting point is the Health Connections page of the website *Race: Are We So Different?* www.understandingrace.org/humvar/biotech.html

Ahmad, W. and Bradby, H. (eds) (2009) *Ethnicity, Health and Health Care. Understanding Diversity, Tacking Disadvantage*. Oxford: Blackwell.

Bradby, H. (2006) 'Racism, ethnicity, biology and society', in A. Clarke and F. Ticehurst (eds) *Living with the Genome. Ethical and Social Aspects of Human Genetics*. Basingstoke: Palgrave. Also at: http://onlinelibrary. wiley.com/doi/10.1002/9780470015902.a0005660/pdf

A variety of publications relevant to this chapter is available from: www. equalityhumanrights.com/about-us/vision-and-mission/our-business-plan/race-equality/

 Online readings

To access further resources related to this chapter, visit the companion website at www.sagepub.co.uk/russell

Atkin, K., Ahmed, S., Hewison, J. and Green, J.M. (2008) 'Decision-making and ante-natal screening for sickle cell and thalassaemia disorders: to what extent do faith and religious identity mediate choice?', *Current Sociology*, 56(1): 77–98.

5

Ageing

Key issues

- The impact of ageing on health is not only a matter of biology
- The ageing process is shaped by social ideas and institutions
- Our health at any particular age reflects the **social construction** of ageing and experiences across our **life course**

Introduction

From a 'common sense' standpoint, ageing might seem a process which is inevitable and biological. Every day we grow older and over time our bodies change. If we live into old age, at some point our major organs will fail and we will die. Yet whilst we tend to think of growing older as a fairly fixed progression of stages, what it means to be any particular age and the condition of our body at that age has much to do with society. This chapter explores what sociology can offer to our understanding of health and ageing. It focuses particularly on old age but also provides a brief discussion of health in childhood and the 'life course' approach to ageing.

A Short History of Ageing

Imagine the kind of life you would associate with a person at the age of one. Imagine the same person at 14, and at 70. The lifestyles we associate with particular ages come from our culture. In other societies, life at different ages was not seen as it is now. For example, in British society children usually have lower status than adults. Amongst the Beng tribe in Africa, however, newborn children are treated with respect because it is believed they have just arrived from the spirit world (Gottlieb, 2004). Whilst in British society older people also have lower status, in traditional Hindu society, a man looks forward to old age. This is the time when his sons will take over support of the family to allow him to devote himself to religious contemplation to assure a better position in the next life. In most societies, women have lower status than men throughout their life (this will be explored further in Chapter 6), but it has usually been in the last part of life that seniority has accorded women the greatest status they will enjoy (Wilson, 2000).

Ideas about the ageing process itself have also evolved over time. In Europe, from ancient times through to the medieval era, it was believed that bodies contained 'radical moisture' and over a lifetime would cool and dry out. For medieval thinkers, health problems, whether in young or older people, related to a variety of external factors and the challenge for all people, regardless of age, was to achieve spiritual goals regardless of the state of the body (Kampf and Botelho, 2009). With the rise of **biomedicine** in the late eighteenth and nineteenth centuries, ageing began to be described in solely biological terms. Old age increasingly came to be characterized in terms of physical decline. A variety of words entered our language which represented ageing in terms of loss and reduced capacity. 'Senescence', for example, is a word that refers to deterioration because of ageing. The biomedical approach to ageing explained old age in terms of internal processes and neglected the impact of a person's wider environment on the state of their bodies over time. It was increasingly assumed that ill health in old age must be related to problems within the ageing body (Katz, 1996).

This new way of thinking about ageing also arose at a time when states were beginning to take much greater interest in monitoring and regulating the lives of citizens. One consequence of this was that age took on a more formal, bureaucratic importance. In most societies, people have not known their birthdays or even their age. Certifying birth became necessary in a society which accorded rights and responsibilities to people at particular ages. We now need 'proof of age' to obtain a driving licence, buy alcohol, have sex, drive a car, marry or obtain age-related benefits when we are older.

Along with these formal age-related rules are a range of associated informal rules which subtly communicate socially constructed ideas about age-appropriate norms and behaviour. Governments, the media, schools and social networks reinforce or revise beliefs that children should not have sex, adults should not live with their parents, men should be older than their female partners, and so on (Vincent, 2003).

A more bureaucratic approach to age had particular implications for older people in society. In Britain, from the sixteenth century, laws known as the Poor Laws regulated institutions which took in people who were poor or vulnerable. These institutions, such as the infamous workhouses, were hardly five-star hotels. Nonetheless, there was no agreement at this time that 'sinners' (which is how the disadvantaged were referred to) had a right to support. It was therefore a great advance when, in the nineteenth century, the Government decided that the poor could be classified into two groups: the 'undeserving' (still seen as sinners) or the 'deserving'. This second group were increasingly viewed as victims of circumstance. Importantly, for older people, the new Poor Law acknowledged that those who had turned 60 fell into this category of the 'deserving' poor. The lives of older people no longer able to work and without families to support them were improved by this development. They now increasingly had a right to a home and food (Laybourne, 1995).

In the twentieth century, the introduction of Old Age Pensions in 1908 gave older people the right to a small income from taxation, and protected them from having to work when they were unable to. Retirement was permitted first at the age of 70 and then, from 1925, at 65 for men, with a retirement age of 60 for women being introduced from 1940 (Thurley, 2013). However, whilst these measures provided some protection for older people, in retrospect this protection came at a cost to their **personhood** (Kitwood, 1997). The lack of autonomy and choice associated with compulsory retirement put older people in a dependent status similar to the status of children. The result was the **infantilization** of older people, which remains a feature of **ageism** towards older people today (Gilleard and Higgs, 2010; Hockey and James, 1993).

Personhood: the status of being counted as a person.

Infantilization: treating a non-infant as if they were an infant.

Shifting Attitudes

However, over the course of the twentieth century, these attitudes came under fire. The context for this shift was the changing age profile of our society. A trend towards people having less children means that we live in a society with an increasingly larger proportion of older people (ONS, 2012c). In addition, life expectancies have increased, from 45 for men and 49 for women around the year 1900 to 78 for men and 82 for women in 2009 (Gjonça et al., 2005: 9/10; ONS, 2011b). By the 1940s, anxieties in Europe and the United States about the growing weight of older people in society led to the fast expansion of gerontology, the 'science of ageing'. Older people themselves fuelled the desire for medical knowledge about the ageing process, wanting science to provide the answers to longevity and even immortality (Kampf and Botelho, 2009).

As people began to live longer, and more of them lived long enough to be able to retire, the desirability of compulsory retirement was called into question. This shift was associated with an important debate amongst sociologists in the 1960s and 1970s. The sociologists Cumming and Henry (1961) viewed retirement as a positive social institution which helped older people to step back from society in preparation for death. They argued that this arrangement was good for society and for the older person themselves. Against this, other sociologists, notably Peter Townsend (who you may remember from Chapter 3), began to argue that forcing people to retire at a fixed age had a negative effect on the health and wellbeing of older people, resulting in enforced or 'structured dependency' (Townsend, 1981). A later generation of sociologists contributed to the development of 'social gerontology'. This school of thought challenged the notion of an automatic link between old age and ill health and highlighted the importance of the social and economic position of people throughout their lives (Tulle-Winton, 1999).

Changes in society and in legislation have therefore been very important for older people, shifting the context in which they have experienced ageing. Like old age, childhood has also changed over time. Industrialized nations, for example, are unique in constructing children as 'innocents'. Social reforms in the nineteenth century constructed children as 'not-yet' people who must be nurtured and trained for society. From the mid-twentieth century, led by the psychologist Jean Piaget, child experts enthusiastically broke childhood down into fixed 'stages' of development by which children worked their way towards competence. Schools are organized on this idea that childhood intellectual development, like physical development, should progress year by year according to age. Encouraged by manufacturers eager to develop new markets, new and previously unknown categories of youth appeared in the latter half of the twentieth century: teenagers, toddlers, young adults and tweenagers (James and Prout, 2005; Rogoff, 2003; Quart, 2003). The following section will consider how the social construction of childhood impacts on the health of children. The chapter will then introduce the influential 'life course' approach to ageing before turning to a detailed examination of the health of older people, commenting briefly on wider attitudes about ageing, and finally, discussing the **sociology** of death and dying.

Childhood and Health

Childhood health patterns today reflect the social construction of childhood and the wider social circumstances of children. There are some health issues associated with young people, which are connected to biological aspects of being young. For example, very young people (similar to those aged 65 and over) are more vulnerable. There are diseases like cystic fibrosis and meningitis which are more associated with the young. Other health problems of children have changed over time. Type 1 diabetes, asthma and obesity, for example, have only recently been on the rise amongst young people (Gale, 2002).

The social circumstances in which children live are crucial to their health patterns. Poorer children are more likely to die before they turn one and more likely to live in an unhealthy environment. They are more likely to have low birth weight or be born prematurely, and more likely to have cerebral palsy, injury, emotional and behavioural problems and to be obese (Howe et al., 2011). It is also in childhood that we learn behaviours that will affect our health as we get older. Growing up in poverty makes a difference to how children eat, how much they exercise, whether they smoke and whether they will breastfeed their own children (Law, 2009). New approaches to the sociology of childhood emphasize, however, that children are not passive in these processes. They play a role in their own wellbeing, developing their competence as health actors in negotiation with significant others. Children, for example, may play a positive role in the family by introducing new health behaviours (James and Prout, 2005).

A Life Course Approach

New approaches to childhood also reflect the influential **life course** approach to thinking about ageing. This approach challenges the idea that stages of life are rooted in biological processes and move in a fixed way from one to the next. It is clear that experiences in early life can shape health across the whole of a person's life. Even in the womb, inadequate nutrition or exposure to dangerous substances can alter organ structures and metabolic functions (Braverman,

2009). In adult life, events such as marrying, having children or retiring have implications for our health. However, these events tend to happen at particular stages of life. Their timing is not fixed. Some transitions in life happen 'on-time', that is, in line with social norms and expectations. Others, due to biology, circumstances or our own choices, may occur 'off-time'. For example, a terminal illness means death comes earlier than expected, unemployment may result in postponing marriage and parenthood, or having a child whilst a teenager might postpone a tertiary education. A life course perspective also means thinking of people as part of a **cohort,** a group of people who are about the same age at the same time. Cohorts share experiences that others cannot. People who were teenagers in the 1960s are different to teenagers today and this has implications for their health experiences (Hutchison, 2007).

> Life course: the sequence of events and activities, reflecting social expectations and institutions, that we encounter as we move from birth through to death.
>
> Cohort: a group of people who share a significant event or experience in a specified time, for example, those born in the same year or decade.

Health in Later Life

Some of us may think about health in later life in fairly negative terms. Old age is often represented as a time when we will be mostly ill or infirm, living in an institution, losing our ability to think clearly. Old age has been associated with being depressed, poor and dependent on others. However, the reality of health for older people is more diverse and complicated than these 'common sense' images suggest.

Most deaths do now occur in old age, compared to earlier times where a variety of dangers meant that most people died 'young'. There are also certain diseases which are more likely to be experienced by older people, such as strokes and dementia. In recent years, there has been fierce debate about whether the 'extra' years achieved by people who are living longer have been years spent in poor health or whether we are living both longer and healthier lives. It is clear that older people are more likely to suffer ill health or disability. For example, in Britain in 2010, 56% of 65 to 74 year olds and 68% of

those aged 75 and over reported a long-standing illness or disability, compared with 19% of 16 to 44 year olds (ONS, 2011a). Nonetheless, these figures also show that 44% of 65 to 74 year olds and about one in three of those
aged 75 and over do *not* suffer from a long-standing illness or disability.

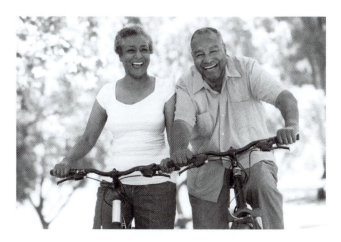

Figure 5.1 Images of older people in advertising material increasingly reflect
social aspirations for healthy ageing

Social scientists also consider which Activities of Daily Living (ADL) a person is able to perform in order to assess how well older people are living. Their
research shows that most older people can perform tasks such as bathing,
climbing stairs and cutting their toenails (Higgs, 2008: 178). So, whilst the
extent of ill health amongst older people, perhaps particularly that minority
classed as 'frail' (Gilleard and Higgs, 2010) may be of concern, it is inaccurate
to imagine that all older people are unwell or incapacitated most of the time.

It is also untrue that older people mostly live in institutions. Less than 10%
of people aged over 65 in developed countries live in any kind of institution,
with most living alone, with their spouse or partner, or with their families.
Amongst those aged over 85 a higher percentage, 20 to 30%, live in some form
of residential care (Wilson, 2000: 19). Nor do most older people suffer from
dementia. The prevalence of dementia in the UK does increase with age, being
suffered by 1.3% of people aged 65 to 69, 12.2% of people aged 80 to 84 and
32.5% of those aged 95 or more. In particular, whilst most people who have
dementia live in the community, more than half of those older people living in
nursing homes and other institutional situations are sufferers (Albanese et al.,
2007: 3–5) (see Case Study: Scottish Dementia Working Group).

Scottish Dementia Working Group

Part of the challenge of improving care for older people is having the sociological imagination to see how improving the circumstances of older people can make a difference to their experience of old age. For people with dementia a major obstacle is the attitudes of other people. The Scottish Dementia Working Group is a group of people with dementia who work together to support one another and help others to better understand dementia. They emphasize that becoming part of an outward-looking group of people facing the same issues and working to improve things for other people with dementia is very empowering. However, other people around them can make life more difficult:

> Losing the ability to work was very disempowering. I felt that if I had been given help to find work which I could still manage I would have felt less disempowered.

> I felt disempowered because the people that spoke to me about dementia always spoke about my loss – all the negative things... they never really took me from the loss of power into the action.

> Some friends take your confidence away. They treat you like a child... People said they would sit me out in the garden as if I was a toy.

> The doctor said to my daughter 'Have you heard of dementia. That's what he's got' and he pointed to me with his thumb.

> We've got to be forceful because professionals can be very patronising. They do their training and they think they have the answers to the world but they need our side of the story.

Source: Scottish Dementia Working Group (2007) *What Disempowers Us – and what can be done.* Glasgow: Alzheimer Scotland.

Whilst dementia is a distressing and common condition amongst older people, nonetheless, even amongst those over 95, it is still suffered by a minority. The focus on dementia may also distract from other mental health issues, in particular, depression (Higgs, 2008), which is the most common mental health issue for older people (Nicholls, 2006). Establishing rates of depression amongst older people is made more difficult because of an assumption that symptoms are just part of getting older. Some suggest only 10–15% of those aged 65 and older and 15% of women and 18% of men aged 80 and over suffer from depression (Evans et al., 2003; McCormick et al., 2009) whilst others find that as many as one in four older people in the community are depressed (Age Concern, 2007).

When older people, perhaps especially those aged 80 and over, do become depressed, this may reflect particular circumstances associated with old age that pose a risk to their emotional wellbeing, notably deteriorating health, the onset of disability, bereavement and relationship breakdown (Banks et al., 2006, cited in McCormick et al., 2009: 5). However, if we consider mental health in general, it is notable that people aged 65 and over suffer significantly less from common mental health problems compared to younger groups (Singleton et al., 2001; ONS, 2010). Running against some of the negative experiences that are more common in old age are an increased ability to cope with loss and disappointment, less vulnerability to persistent negative moods compared with young adults, more resistance to criticism and a greater ability to control and balance emotions (Carstensen, 2009, cited in McCormick et al., 2009: 4). Nonetheless, older people in institutions in particular are more vulnerable to mental ill health, which goes unrecognized or undetected (Hsu et al., 2005). There are also a number of rarer mental health problems that affect older people specifically, such as delirium, anxiety and late-onset schizophrenia (Mental Health Foundation, 2012).

Old Age and Poverty

Another image of older people associates old age with poverty. Yet older people are neither more nor less likely to be poor. In Britain, pensioner incomes have grown over the last 30 years, with the result that age is not a strong predictor of hardship (Middleton, 2007). Indeed, in some European countries (though not in Britain), risk of poverty decreases with age (Naegele and Walker in Bond et al., 2007: 148). The late twentieth century saw an important shift in the lifestyles and opportunities of many older people, leading the theorist Peter Laslett (1989) to suggest that retirement could potentially mean, not the end to productive involvement in society, but the beginning of an exciting new 'third age' of opportunity, good health and personal development (Gilleard and Higgs, 2002). The proportion of pensioners who are in the bottom fifth of households in terms of net income after housing costs decreased since 1979 from 43% to 13% in 2010–11, a dramatic improvement (DWP, 2011: 66).

However, not all older people are enjoying the same improvement. Whilst some are in a comfortable position, some of the poorest people in British society are old. Older people who are more vulnerable to poverty include women, especially widows, those over 75, people who lived on low incomes during their working lives and ethnic minority people (DWP, 2011; Naegele and Walker in Bond et al., 2007). Much evidence indicates that someone whose life and work has been hard on their health will find that hardship 'written on the body' in old age. The negative effects of long-term exposure to bad environments accumulate and are more important for life expectancy than factors like smoking or exercise (Bartley and Blane, 2009).

Interdependence

Older people can also be portrayed both as lonely and lacking connection with other people yet simultaneously as dependent on others. A more useful way to think about this is to recognize the interdependence of all human beings and the way patterns of interdependence change as we age. It is true that because the chance of continuing to live with a spouse decreases as a person ages, many older people live alone. For example, in 2010 around 25% of British people aged 65 to 74 and over 45% of those aged 75 and over lived alone (ONS, 2011b).

However, as these statistics show, whilst many older people live alone, most do not. Moreover, living alone is not the same thing as being lonely. Older people are not more lonely than other age groups, despite the 'persistent sterotype of the inevitability of loneliness in later life' (Victor et al., 2009: 224). Most older people have children or siblings living close to them with whom they are in frequent contact as they are with friends and neighbours with whom they maintain strong and enduring relationships (Victor et al., 2009). A study of older people in Wales noted that the process of replacing friends continues on into very old age (Jerrome and Wenger, 1999, cited in Askham et al. in Bond et al., 2007: 194). Older people also show high levels of commitment to local communities through volunteering and participation in local groups (Victor et al., 2009: 224).

Ageism

Some of the most important problems faced by older people have nothing to do with physical decline. The **2010 Equality Act** requires public bodies like the NHS to take action to ensure that ageism does not result in unequal treatment for any of their service users, as they do to redress institutional racism (see Chapter 4) and gender inequality (to be discussed in Chapter 6). However, unequal treatment in health care due to age does occur. Some of this unequal treatment affects young people. Evidence suggests, for example, that those aged 16 to 17 receive less favourable treatment from health services, perhaps especially mental health services, than adults or younger children (Young Equals, 2009: 8). In relation to

Table 5.1 Percentage of respondents observing ageist activity

Statement	Sometimes or often	Rarely, sometimes or often
Not being referred to specialist services locally or outside the area when this is needed	42	79
Older people having a low priority with respect to medical attention, referrals, surgery or investigation	37	84
Not being referred for investigations such as blood test, x-rays or scans	34	71
Having difficulty getting some services to see a person who is over 65	29	66
Not having surgery despite being fit enough	21	63
Not having cardiac investigations or treatments such as pacemakers because of age	18	53
Being excluded from respite care because you are over 65, even if you had it before	16	45
Not being offered the chance to take part in research, such as entering a clinical trial	16	34
Having difficulty getting on to a GP list	13	47
Having problems getting a recuperative care bed if you are over 65	13	47

n=57 (Billings, 2003)

Source: Lievesley, N. (2009) *Ageism and age discrimination in secondary health care in the United Kingdom. A Review from the Literature*. London: Centre for Policy on Ageing, Department of Health: 17

older people there is much evidence that despite the increasing need of older people for adequate health care, discrimination and unsatisfactory care are extremely common (Lievesley et al., 2009: 8) (see Table 5.1).

In everyday medical practice doctors routinely make decisions about how best to use resources and deal with waiting lists with an agenda that older people are less worthy of help (Bond and Cabrero in Bond et al., 2007: 118). The idea that ill health is 'normal' and even inevitable for older people also often results in unsatisfactory care (see Case Study: Nursing Students' Attitudes to Ageing Service Users). Research in the 1990s found social workers spent less time and had fewer contacts with older oncology patients than younger patients (Rohan et al., 1994, cited in Minichiello et al., 2000: 254). Depression amongst older people can go unaddressed by health and social care practitioners who view depression as a 'normal' aspect of ageing (Age Concern, 2007).

Ageism: discrimination based on a person's age.

CASE STUDY

Nursing Students' Attitudes to Ageing Service Users

The quality of health care received by older people who are unwell or suffering from dementia is crucial to their wellbeing. A number of Australian researchers have interviewed student nurses about their attitudes to older people and found that there are significant obstacles to this quality care being provided. Wendy Moyle (2003) found 10% of students she interviewed in Australia believed people over 65 should be forced into retirement to make positions available for younger people. She found students imagined old age in negative, stereotyped ways and said they did not want to work in aged care because they saw it as depressing (Moyle, 2003: 19). Students interviewed at the very beginning of their training said it would be sad working with old people and it was perceived that old people are simply 'waiting to die' (Henderson et al., 2008). Many respondents said that they did not like older people and found them difficult to communicate with and hard to relate to. De la Rue (2003), speaking to final year nursing students, found that they feared the ageing process and Robinson and Cubit (2005) found this fear was associated with distaste for and discomfort with older bodies. Whilst Henderson found that students who had experience working with older people were more positive about working with older people, other evidence suggests that as students spend more time in aged care their negative attitudes may instead be reinforced. Koh (2012) notes that British students share similar attitudes and need to be better prepared for the realities of caring for older people, which may leave them feeling overwhelmed, scared and intimidated.

Sources: Moyle, W. (2003) 'Nursing student's perceptions of older people: continuing society's myth', *Australian Journal of Advanced Nursing*, 20(4): 15–21; Henderson, J., Xiao, L., Siegloff, L., Kelton, M. and Paterson, J. (2008) ' "Older people have lived their lives": first year nursing students' attitudes towards older people', *Contemporary Nurse*, 30: 32–45; de la Rue, M. (2003) 'Preventing ageism in nursing students: an action theory approach', *Australian Journal of Advanced Nursing*, 20(4): 8–14; Robinson, A. and Cubit, K. (2005) 'Student nurses' experiences of the body in aged care', *Contemporary Nurse*, 19: 41–51; Koh, L.C. (2012) 'Student attitudes and educational support in caring for older people – a review of literature', *Nurse Education in Practice*, 12(1): 16–20.

One consequence of ageism is that older people internalize messages that they are of less value than younger people. Surveys of people aged 65 and older in 2000/1 found 37% said that if they were about to receive cardiac surgery they would be willing to swap places with a person aged 45 who was six months behind them on the waiting list (Lievesley, 2009: 15). Older people may also hold negative beliefs about their own ageing which affect their ability to stay healthy. They may expect symptoms and therefore fail to mention these to their doctor, even when there are treatments that might help them (Bond and Cabrero in Bond et al., 2007: 116/7). As the movement for healthy or successful ageing has highlighted, much evidence indicates that many physical problems of older people are the result of lifestyle factors such as diet and a lack of exercise (Kendig and Browning, 2010).

A Society Obsessed by Ageing?

Today, there are more older people than ever before. Whilst some evidence suggests this creates potential for rifts between the young and the old, there are many similarities in the challenges facing both groups. Ageing is also no longer just the concern of older people. Enthusiasm for buying products to alter our appearance and keep ourselves 'young' increasingly preoccupies younger people (Gilleard and Higgs, 2000). Our consumer culture offers many ways for us to spend money to ward off the effects of ageing, whether in our appearance or in our physical capabilities, including anti-wrinkle creams, botox, cosmetic surgery and replacement hips and knees. There has been a powerful drive to develop medical technology to prolong life or enhance its quality in old age. In the US, for example, people in their eighties are the most rapidly growing group of surgical patients (Kaufman et al., 2004: 3). In a society which values individual identity it is not surprising that there are also fierce debates about the extent to which medicine will be able to extend the life span (Vincent, 2006, 2009).

Twenty-first century changes to the law protect older people from compulsory retirement, facilitating their greater economic independence. Like the movement of many more women into the workforce after the Second World War (which will be discussed in the next chapter), this change has been controversial for some. However, the greater independence of older people is of benefit to society as a whole, not just the old. In addition to the contributions they have made to taxation over the course of their working lives, older people currently contribute many hours of unpaid labour into the economy. Research commissioned in 2011 found people over 65 contributed £40billion to the British economy in 2010 through taxes, spending, provision of social care, volunteering and other contributions and this is set to increase substantially (WRVS, 2011). Whilst older people do make more use of health services, including more expensive health care, this cost is mainly due to the expense of care in the very last months of a person's life, which is high for anyone who is dying, regardless of how old they are (Wanless, 2002).

Death and Dying

Our anxieties and concerns about ageing are closely related to concerns about death. In our society, death is seen as a very negative event, but this is not universal. There are many societies in which praying daily for death to come soon is a normal way to approach the end of life (Wilson, 2000). Death can occur at any age, but it is the inevitable endpoint of old age, and in our society, an increasing proportion of people will not die until they are old (Seale, 2000).

Like ageing, death has certain unalterable physiological characteristics but there is much about it that is cultural. Where once, the moment of death was judged through the loss of a pulse, medical advances have given us the concept of 'brain death', where blood can continue to pump through the body after the nerve centre has ceased to function (Timmermans, 2000). Today, we view death as a medical process. Despite a trend in recent decades towards caring for dying people in the community, death usually happens in a hospital. Most people do not die suddenly but are unwell before they die and only enter hospital at the end. A minority will die in a hospice (especially people who die from cancer) or some other institution.

Because of the **medicalization** of death, most of us, at the very end of our lives, are likely to be in close contact with health care professionals. Since most of the care of the dying is undertaken by unpaid relatives, relationships between doctors, nurses and relatives, therefore, are likely to be important to what kind of experience dying will be. Awareness that life is likely to have a 'medical' end has resulted in the rise of 'living wills', legal documents created by individuals to exert some control over decisions made by medical professionals and others that will impact on the nature of their death.

As suggested in Chapter 2, we live in an individualistic society in which a moral life involves making responsible choices about our own health, nutrition and lifestyle. When we have worked to stay healthy all our lives death may seem like some kind of failure, not only for us but for others who have tried to keep us healthy. For biomedicine, death represents the limits of the reach of science, limits which anti-ageing science still aspires to overcome (Vincent, 2006, 2009). One feature of our society is a rising proportion of people suffering chronic illness (see Chapter 8) and hospice care increasingly involves short-term management of often unpleasant symptoms such as a loss of bodily functions. It has been suggested that this profoundly distressing experience, in a society that sees bodily self control as essential to personhood, may shake a person's very sense of being a person (Lawton, 2000).

The care provided by health and social care professionals therefore involves not only physical help with bodily degeneration associated with dying, but support for individuals and those close to them as they try to work out how to live and think about their life as it nears its end. Whilst traditional approaches were concerned with professional openness to help the dying and their family 'come to terms' with death, sociologists of dying have highlighted the uncertainty of the dying process, even when the end is close and inevitable, and even after it has occurred. The dying person may continue to have significance long after they have died as a positive presence in the daily routines of those whose lives they were part of (Bowling and Cartwright, 1982).

Implications for Practice

In the past, health and social care has frequently been delivered in light of 'common sense' ideas about age and judgements about what is possible and appropriate support for people at particular ages: 'she is too young to know what's best for her'; 'he can't expect improvement at his age'. Health and social care practice has reflected the medicalization of the processes both of ageing and dying. However, recent trends emphasize the personhood of people and the importance of supporting their right to actively make their own decisions about their health and wellbeing throughout their lives, including when their lives are ending. In this, health care professionals have a crucial role to play.

Summary

- Youth, old age and dying are social as well as biological experiences
- The health and wellbeing of most older people is different from the 'common sense' views that are held about them
- Our capacity to be competent and to care for ourselves may be helped or hindered by social constructions of ageing

Exercise

1. Have you ever had the experience of being 'judged' because of your age? Have you ever been with someone who has been treated differently because of their age?
2. What are some ways age discrimination might lead to a service user receiving inadequate care in your profession?

Further Reading

Bond, J., Peace, S.M., Dittmann-Kohli, F. and Westerhof, G. (2007) *Ageing in Society: An Introduction to Social Gerontology*. Third edition. London: Sage.

Higgs, P. and Rees Jones, I. (2008) *Medical Sociology and Old Age. Towards a Sociology of Health in Later Life*. London: Routledge.

Vincent, J.A. (2003) *Old Age*. Key Ideas Series. London: Routledge.

Students interested in learning more about the mental health of older people, will find the Social Care Institute for Excellence suite of online modules a useful introduction. Available at: www.scie.org.uk/publications/elearning/mentalhealth/index.asp

 ## Online readings

To access further resources related to this chapter, visit the companion website at www.sagepub.co.uk/russell

Vincent, J. A. (2006) 'Ageing contested: anti-ageing science and the cultural construction of old age', *Sociology*, 40: 681–98.

6

Gender

Key issues

- Differences between men and women are not simply the product of biology but are socially constructed
- These **gender** differences have an important impact on our health
- The different ways that gender impacts on the health of men and women are complex

Introduction

One of the first things a child learns about itself, in our society, is whether they are a boy or a girl. If we are **intersex**, that is, one of the 1.7% of people whose sex may be difficult to categorize as male or female when we are born (Krane and Barak, 2012: 39; Moore, 2000), this is likely to be a source of anxiety for our parents; should they dress the baby in pink or blue? The child *must* be one or the other (more about intersexuality in Chapter 7). From infancy onwards, our gender seems fundamental to the kind of person we are. The 'common sense' view of gender suggests that the characteristics that go with being a boy or a girl are laid down in our genes. By this account, we develop into men and

women due to fixed biological processes that shape not only the development of our bodies but of our personalities, including who we are
attracted to sexually. Whilst ideas about the relative abilities of men and
women have changed over recent decades, most people still see gender
as a fairly fixed aspect of who we are. However, gender, like **social class**,
ethnicity and the experience of ageing, is socially constructed. This chapter will explore the social construction of gender difference and what
gender means for the health of women and men.

Intersex: someone whose sex may be difficult to categorize as male or
female due to ambiguous genitalia or other biological characteristics.

Gender: an aspect of identity that we make when we act or speak in
ways that show our sense of what it means to be male or female in our
society.

A Short History of Gender Difference

Until the twentieth century, in most societies, women had less status
than men. Their everyday lives and responsibilities reflected that lower
status. Women were also not usually in positions of power in society
and it was usually, on the whole, better to be born male. Women had
very low status in ancient Greek society, for example. Nonetheless, the
lives of men and women do not look the same in every society we can
consider. There are many examples of societies where ideas about **masculinities** and **femininities** are quite different to those we are familiar
with. Traditional native American tribes, for example, have embraced
individuals known as Two-Spirits, people who do not conform to femininity or masculinity as we know them. Two-Spirits speak and behave
in ways that we might associate with men or women. They do not identify as heterosexual or gay, nor do they consider themselves **transgender**,
but they may have sexual relationships with people of the same gender
(Walters et al., 2011).

Masculinities and femininities: ways of speaking and behaving that reflect socially constructed ideas about what it means to be male or female.

Transgender: someone who does not easily fit into the social norm whereby people are seen as being born either male or female and as having particular desires, personalities and behaviours biologically fixed by their sex.

In most societies, however, there have been strong cultural differences between men and women, which mostly disadvantaged women. The first real challenge to inequality between the sexes dates to the nineteenth century. As discussed in previous chapters, in Western Europe the nineteenth century was a time of great change. This century saw the rise of a new social system and the dominance of science and reason as a way of understanding the world. In addition, some **Enlightenment** thinkers argued that the new ideal of equality for all should extend to women.

From the eighteenth century onwards, however, doctors, the vast majority male, resisted this trend and built a body of evidence which portrayed women as biologically inferior to men, physically weaker, less intelligent and more emotionally vulnerable by nature. In this, they were moving away from a view many centuries old of men's and women's bodies as being essentially similar. The ancient Greeks, for example, believed that men's and women's genitals were essentially the same organs, but on the outside for men and on the inside for women (Laqueur, 1990). By the nineteenth century, **biomedicine** viewed men and women as fundamentally different, physically, emotionally and intellectually. The diagnosis of 'hysteria', for example, was used to describe women who did not focus their energies on marriage and child-bearing but on pursuing education and a career. It was believed that emotional problems and even infertility would result if the womb was not used for its supposedly biologically intended purpose (having children) (Scull, 2009). Late in the nineteenth century, the admission of women to university was resisted on the grounds that menstruation made women too delicate for academic work (Talairach-Vielmas, 2007: 34).

For decades, a minority of women struggled for greater equality for women. An important turning point for their efforts was the Second World War. As industries were forced to take on women to replace the men who were away fighting, people began to see that perhaps women could play other roles in society in addition to raising children. In the long economic boom that followed, more and more women became wage-earners (as well as taking main responsibility for child care at home). The changing lives of women were accompanied by shifts in the way people thought about women's personalities and abilities, and they also changed the way we think about men. From being relatively fixed in the past, our sense of what it means to be male or female has changed enormously in a generation or two, and continues to evolve.

The Social Construction of Gender

Sociologists have found it useful to make a distinction between the idea of **sex** and gender. Sex refers to the differences between male and female bodies, whereas gender refers to differences which reflect social norms. Much research has explored the ways we learn how to behave according to our gender. Gender gets made and re-made because we are born into a world which is gendered (Blaise, 2005; Paechter, 2007). From the time that we are identified as male or female in infancy, we can observe all around us clues about how to 'do' gender. Gender is on display for us in the ways people identified as male and female behave; we see it in how they dress, how they speak, even how they move. As children we soon begin to demonstrate our sense about what gender means for us through the kind of toys we choose to play with, the colours we prefer, and the way that we experience our bodies, for example, our experiences of hunger (see Case Study: Learning to Eat Like a Boy or a Girl). The family, media, school and the workplace are some of the areas where gender is on display and where we can be gently or even harshly reminded if we 'do' gender in the 'wrong' way.

> Sex: whether a person has the anatomical characteristics normally associated with men or women.

Learning to Eat Like a Boy or a Girl

Eating disorders, both those associated with under- and over-eating, are features of modern society about which there has been much comment. Whilst both men and women struggle with over-weight, women are more likely to be under-weight than men. Many writers have linked women's eating problems to the social pressures on women to be slim. Researchers Jill Holm-Denoma et al. were interested to know how mothers and fathers viewed the body size and shape of their boy and girl children and what messages they were communicating to them about how they should eat. They surveyed parents of children of identical BMI. They found that whilst parents did not describe their children's body size and shape differently for boys and girls, they did report eating behaviours differently. Whilst boys and girls in the sample were equally 'picky', fathers noticed their sons refusing food more than mothers did. Mothers also reported that their daughters were eating enough but that their sons weren't. Both mothers and fathers were more likely to worry that their sons but not their daughters were underweight. Mothers were also more likely to comment if their daughters had good appetites (but did not comment about this in relation to their sons). These findings support the theory that there are different body ideals for boys and girls, with girls receiving greater encouragement to appear thin and not overeat. It appears that parents may unintentionally communicate these expectations even to very young children.

Source: Holm-Denoma, J.M. (2005) 'Parents' reports of the body shape and feeding habits of 36-month-old children: an investigation of gender differences', *International Journal of Eating Disorders,* 28(3): 228–35.

A minority of us, despite this subtle and not-so-subtle training, do break gender norms. For example, people who identify as gay, are those who, despite receiving many messages from society that say they should only be attracted people of the 'opposite' sex, experience their bodies and their desires in a different way. The existence of gay and transgendered people highlights that to understand gender, we need to speak of masculinities and femininities, not just males and females. Our gender is social constructed and there are more than two options available to us. A useful concept to help think about this is **'hegemonic masculinity'**. This idea highlights that there are different types of masculinity. Heterosexual masculinity is the dominant, socially acceptable form of masculinity ('hegemonic' means predominant). People who conform to this type of masculinity are rewarded by society. They have better access to power and status in society. Women are one group obviously disadvantaged by this kind of 'gender order'. However, some men are also disadvantaged by it. For example, 'real' men are not supposed to cry in public, and a man who does cry in public will receive subtle messages from others watching that this is not a very 'manly' way to behave. Those who in various ways don't or can't conform to these informal rules, including gay and transgender people, face discrimination and stigma for not following the hegemonic masculine norms (Connell and Messerschmidt, 2005).

> Hegemonic masculinity: the way of 'doing' gender that is most valued in our society (the best people are the ones who can 'be a man').

Gender Inequality in the UK

What does the social construction of gender mean for our patterns of health and illness? An important place to start is to acknowledge the extent to which women are still disadvantaged in society. It is common today to hear the belief expressed that the women's movement has mostly achieved its aims. Women have been allowed to vote for nearly a century. We are no longer legally a possession of our husbands, excluded from most occupations and rarely seen in high status positions in society. However, unfortunately, statistics show equality is still some way off. Women are still seen as naturally best suited to looking after children and performing domestic and 'emotional' tasks, both in the family and in society. Moreover, this kind of work is not financially rewarded, precisely because, as 'women's work', it is not valued in the way that 'men's work' is valued.

Women's inequality has implications for health, so it is important to establish the reality of this inequality. One of the obstacles to recognizing it has been the difficulty of measuring the social position of women. For example, until fairly recently, measures used to compare **social class** were designed to measure differences between men and did not work well for measuring women's **socio-economic** situation. The Registrar General's classification/scale (shown in Table 3.1 in Chapter 3) classified both men and women according to the occupation of the 'head of household' – the man. Today, women's socio-economic position is measured by considering a number of factors such as 'education, housing tenure, occupation, income,

absolute or relative material wealth, and area-based measures of deprivation'
(Hunt and Batty, 2009: 146).

One key marker of health status is whether or not a person has paid employment and studies confirm that paid work is good for both physical and mental
health (Gabe et al., 2004: 13; Bartley et al., 1992; Bradby, 2008). This has
implications for any man or woman unable to work for any reason, but women
are more likely to be without work. Whilst the gap has narrowed due to women
having children later and older mothers being more likely to work, in 2011,
35.4% of women compared to 5.7% of men were economically inactive
because they were looking after family or home. The employment rate for men
in 2010 was 10% higher than for women (ONS, 2011b).

In addition, women are also far more likely than men to work part-time
(Annandale, 2009: 113) and much part-time work is poorly paid. Hence,
jobs held by women are more likely to fall below the minimum wage. Though
it has been illegal for some decades to pay a woman less money for the same
job as a man, the concentration of women in less well-paid occupations and
in part-time posts mean that the average full-time wage of a woman in Britain
is 14.9% of the average man's and for part-time work, 9.1% (ONS, 2012d).
Women who have children must juggle both paid work and unpaid work in
the home, as work undertaken in the home continues to be conducted mainly
by women. For example, eight out of ten married women in British households still do more housework than their husbands (IPPR, 2012). Women
are more likely to spend a larger amount of their time, over the course of
their lives, caring for other people: preparing food for them, cleaning for
them and helping them organize their lives.

These patterns in women's lives all result in women being more vulnerable
to poverty. This vulnerability increases as we age. Over the course of a woman's life, she will have less opportunity than a man to save for retirement,
particularly if, like most women, she has any children and has to leave the
workforce when they are small. In addition, women are less likely to have
paid national insurance over the whole of their working life time and/or to
have contributed to a pension. This is why the 'gender gap' in pay between
men and women grows substantially after the age of 39 (ONS, 2012d).

Men Die Quicker but Women get Sicker?

It might be tempting to conclude from this discussion of women's inequality
that women would be more vulnerable to ill health than men. To some
extent, this may be true. However, class differences and a variety of other

factors mean that the differences between men and women in terms of their health are surprisingly complicated. The first and most simple example of this can be seen when we consider differences in mortality (death) and morbidity (illness). Despite the disadvantages of being female in our society, since the twentieth century, women in Britain have lived longer, on average, than men. Around 1900, men could expect to live to about 45 and women to 49. By 1950 the average age of death was 66.5 for males and 71.3 for females (Gjonça et al., 2005: 9/10). By 2009 life expectancy for men was 78.1 years and for females, 82.1 years (ONS, 2011b). That is, women now live, on average, four years longer than men in Britain.

In the past, this was a puzzle for sociologists, since much evidence shows that women are more vulnerable to ill health. In Britain and similar countries, women experience more chronic but not necessarily life-threatening illness and disability than men. As a consequence, it is often said that the extra years of life enjoyed by women (because they live longer) are typically not spent in good health (Annandale, 2009: 58). In recent years, the quality of life of people at the end of their lives is now taken into account. Statisticians now consider, in addition to life expectancy, 'healthy life expectancy' (the number of years a person can expect to live in good health) and 'disability-free life expectancy' (Wood et al., 2006). In 2008–10, the healthy life expectancy for men and women in the UK was very similar: 63.5 years for men and 65.7 for women (you can learn more about these measures from an ONS clip available in the website that goes with this book).

Why would women be sicker if it is men who die quicker? On closer inspection, the data suggests a complex picture behind the different rates of mortality and morbidity for men and women. In countries like Britain the major factor in the improvement in life expectancy for men and women after 1930 was a fall in infant mortality rates (ONS, 2011b). More and more people surviving infancy meant that when the average length of life was calculated, the figure gradually increased over the years. More recently, life expectancy is increasing because of falls in the rate of deaths due to cancer, heart and circulatory disease (ONS, 2011b). However, there are more men than women surviving these diseases, and as a result the 'gap' between the length of life of men and women is disappearing (Annandale and Field, 2007: 100).

Seen in a wider context, it is clear that the length of life of men and women is not fixed and depends on circumstances. Until 1930, for example, men in Britain lived on average a little longer than women (Gjonça et al., 2005: 10). Prior to that, many girls aged 5 to 15 died from infectious and parasitic diseases, especially tuberculosis, partly due to the conditions in which they were living. Women now outlive men in all countries, but this is quite recent.

The improvements that lengthened the lives of women in countries like Britain are only now coming about in the majority world, where childbirth in particular remains a major killer (Barford et al., 2006).

Just as mortality rates have become more similar, it appears that some differences in morbidity between men and women are also decreasing. If we consider GP records of consultation rates (how many men make appointments and how many women) it is clear that, on the whole, women consult more than men. Biological factors seem to be the most important factor in this, since consulting rates differ most for the ages when women are in their reproductive years. In 2009 6% of women and 4% of men attended a GP consultation but between the ages of 16 and 44 women were twice as likely to visit. However, if we compare records of self-reported health, in recent years these have suggested only a very small difference between men and women, except amongst people aged over 65 (ONS, 2011b).

The debate about whether 'men die quicker but women get sicker' illustrates that the health patterns of men and women are too complicated to be summed up simply and neatly. Partly this is because people who share a gender may be very different from one another in other ways, because of their social class, ethnicity, age, sexuality or nationality. Nonetheless, gender inequalities and the social ideal of hegemonic masculinity mean that there are particular health issues associated with being identified as male or female which are always tied up with the kinds of lives that are expected for men and women. The following sections offer some insight into these issues by considering, first, the health of women, second, the health of men, and finally, how gender makes a difference to two important behaviours which are detrimental for health, drinking and smoking.

Women's Health

It is obvious that some important women's health problems relate to having a female body. Most notably, in one part of their lives, most women may become pregnant and have a baby, whereas men may not. Many health problems are associated with female reproductive functions. Other problems are very obviously not about female bodies but about the kinds of lives that women live in our society. Many studies have shown that the domestic responsibilities usually associated with women can have a negative impact on both physical and mental health (Doyal, 1995). Motherhood and child care also results in a lack of control for women over their own needs. Women see themselves as responsible for caring and so put the needs of the family first, tending to subjugate their own needs in terms of income, food and so on, and ultimately, their own health, to the needs of others (Popay and Jones, 1991).

The higher levels of depression and anxiety reported by women have been explained in part by reference to women's work in caring for others with what may be insufficient amounts of time, money and other resources. This is especially true for those women raising and caring for their families in poverty. There is also evidence that changes to women's roles, though improving life in some ways, have in other ways added to women's workload, creating a 'double burden'. Nettleton (1995) argued that women may suffer more illness because they have to undertake more social roles than men, and the nature and quality of these multiple roles are likely to be detrimental to their health. In a society that values physical strength and devalues those who are less strong, women are also more vulnerable to violence (see Case Study: Intimate Partner Violence Against Women).

CASE STUDY

Intimate Partner Violence Against Women: The Health Costs

In recent years intimate partner violence has been identified by the World Health Organization as a major human rights and health issue. A review of research up to 1999 in 35 countries revealed that 10–52% of women reported being physically abused at some point in their lives by an intimate partner, with 10–30% experiencing sexual violence. This violence carries a considerable health cost. For example, a 2006 study in Victoria, Australia, found that amongst women of reproductive age, partner violence accounted for 7.9% of the overall disease burden to women, being a larger risk to health than blood pressure, tobacco use and increased body weight. A 2012 study revealed that in most countries surveyed, women who had experienced violence at the hands of their partners were significantly more likely to report poor or very poor health. They were also more likely to have had problems with walking and carrying out daily activities, pain, memory loss, dizziness and vaginal discharge in the four weeks prior to the interview. Women who had ever been abused by their partners also experienced significantly higher levels of emotional distress. There are also a variety of indirect costs. For example, a woman who has been injured by her partner may struggle to work or study, affecting the whole family's socio-economic circumstances. Training for health care professionals to learn to identify women experiencing violence at home is lacking, as is follow-up care and protection.

Sources: Garcia-Moreno, C. and Watts, C. (2011) 'Editorial: Violence against women: an urgent public health priority', *Bull World Health Organ*, 89(2): 2–3; Gracia-Moreno, C.

et al. (2012) *WHO Multi-Country Study on Women's Health and Domestic Violence Against Women. Initial Results on Prevalence, Health Outcomes and Women's Responses. Summary Report.* Geneva: World Health Organization.

There are also a number of behaviours associated with feminine norms which have negative health implications, particularly in relation to the extra emphasis that is still placed on women's appearance as a source of personal value. The pressure put on women to live up to the 'Beauty Myth' (Wolf, 1991) has been associated with eating disorders linked to poor body image, unnecessary cosmetic surgery and self-harm (Hepp et al., 2005) (see Figure 6.1).

The lower value of women in society can be reflected in differential treatment in health care. In the majority world, differences in availability and quality of reproductive health care in particular have an impact on the length of life of women (Hunt and Batty, 2009: 143, citing Doyal et al., 2001). In developed countries, strategies for investigation and treatment of disease have been shown to be different for men and women and doctors interpret symptoms differently and use different conversation styles with male and female patients (Malterud and Okkes, 1998: 404). Arber et al. (2006, cited in Annandale and Field, 2007: 106) presented a set of case studies to doctors in the UK and US and told the doctors some were female and some were

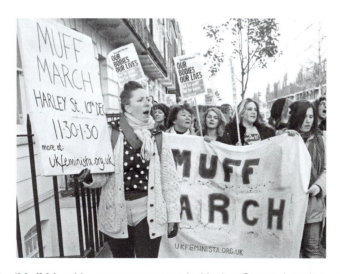

Figure 6.1 'Muff March' – women protest in Harley Street, London, about the increase in demand for 'designer vagina' cosmetic surgery, December, 2011
Photograph by Alan Denney

male. They found women were asked fewer questions, given fewer examina-
tions and tests and were prescribed less medication, with women in 'midlife'
being asked the least questions and prescribed the least medication. Services
specifically for women also tend to focus on reproductive issues. This is
good for women in a particular age group, but means that the health problems of women who have not become or are no longer fertile are relatively
neglected (Afifi, 2007: 386).

This example highlights that there are particular issues associated with
ageing for women. Having survived infancy, boys and girls have very
similar health profiles (Gabe et al., 2004) but differences emerge later,
providing support for the importance of social context and gendered
lives for many sex differences in health. During and after menopause, for
example, women suffer from a distinctive discrimination, which is not
just about gender nor age, but about the particular way our society has
treated women who can no longer have children. From ancient times
onwards, women who are no longer fertile have been subject to a variety
of negative stereotypes. Older women, therefore, face particular challenges
(Macdonald, 2002).

Men's Health

As for women, some health problems suffered by men result from having a
male body. Before and shortly after birth, male babies are more likely to die.
Premature birth, cerebral palsy, congenital malformation and Sudden Infant
Death Syndrome are all more common amongst boys. In addition, coronary
heart disease (CHD), a major killer of both men and women, starts earlier
in men and evidence suggests that the female hormone oestrogen may protect women before menopause (Annandale and Field, 2007: 94). Statistically, the result of more male babies dying and of men dying younger from
CHD is to reduce the average life expectancy of men.

Other problems relate to the kind of lives men live in our society.
Hegemonic masculinity results in inequality for women but it also causes
problems for men. This may relate to the kind of work men do. For
example, a study of debt collectors found that men in this job are
required to be routinely aggressive, a stance which affects their relationship with their bodies (Hochschild, 1983). Masculinity has been implicated in CHD (Elmslie and Hunt, 2009) and in higher rates of male
death in motor vehicle accidents and accidents associated with risky leisure
activities (Creighton and Oliffe, 2010; Schmid Mast et al., 2008; Courtenay,
2000). It is men who fight in wars with two world wars in the twentieth

century having a major impact on male mortality rates (Gjonça et al., 2005: 11). These behaviours are culturally based and not the product of male biology. One indication of this is the rise of more risky leisure patterns amongst young women, again reflecting changing cultural norms (Lumsden, 2010).

It has also been suggested that gender 'norms' are bad for men because they are more inclined to 'suffer in silence' when they are unwell. For example, one study found that men who strongly endorse hegemonic masculinity are 46% less likely to obtain preventative health services (Springer and Mouzon, 2011). As Courtenay has argued:

> The most powerful men among men are those for whom health and safety are irrelevant... When a man brags, "I haven't been to a doctor in years", he is simultaneously describing a health practice and situating himself in a masculine arena (Courtenay, 2000: 1389) (see Case Study).

It has been suggested that it is more difficult for men to seek help and that this may explain differences in consultation rates between women and men and other factors, such as the higher suicide rates of men (Barr et al., 2012).

. . . .

'I'm hard, I'm daft, I'll cut my arm off and just grow another one back': Masculinity and Help Seeking

Researchers in Glasgow wanted to explore what men had to say about their willingness to seek help in relation to health problems, and to find out how this related to their ideas about masculinity and what it means to be a man. They ran focus groups with men aged 15–74 from a variety of backgrounds and occupations. What they found was that young men in particular emphasized that they would not go to the doctor unless the problem was serious. The episodes the men chose to talk about also tended to involve situations where they had been hurt being 'manly': 'the only time I have (gone) to hospital or seen a doctor... was when I had been punched in the face (and)... I needed stitches...' Asked to explain why they would not seek help until the problem was serious, one man said: 'You don't like to make a fuss because it's a macho thing just to say you're being the strong silent type... You'll endure it, you can take it'. The men interviewed saw being able to withstand pain as a sign of their masculinity, agreeing that men 'should be able to push things further'. This was seen as a way of distinguishing themselves from women: 'If a woman cut themselves they'd be away to the doctor. A guy'd be like "I'll just go and get myself a bit of Sellotape and wrap it up"'. Men from the Asian Group surveyed emphasized

CASE STUDY

(Continued)

(Continued)

the emotional self-sufficiency of men: 'the more masculine man... can sort it out himself... He doesn't need anyone else'.

Source: O'Brien R. et al. (2005) ' "It's caveman stuff, but that is to a certain extent how guys still operate": Men's accounts of masculinity and help seeking', *Social Science and Medicine*, 61: 503–16.

....

However, whilst this image of the 'stoic' man is a popular explanation for gender differences in health, some studies cast doubt on the idea that, unlike men, women find it easy to admit to problems and ask for help. Interviews with 10-, 13- and 15-year-old boys and girls in Scotland, for example, have highlighted that both boys and girls can be reluctant to seek help for symptoms, especially psychological ones (MacLean et al., 2010).

Drinking, Smoking and Gender

Feminine and masculine norms are also relevant to mortality differences linked to drinking and smoking (McCartney, 2011). Alcohol, for example, has been implicated in many medical conditions including cancer, hypertensive disease, cirrhosis and depression. Alcohol-related deaths amongst men have been increasing since 1991, especially amongst men living in deprived areas. Rates of alcohol-related death for women, however, have been declining. Whilst rates of consumption have been decreasing for both men and women since 2002, heavy drinking is traditionally a male pastime. For example, since 1979, roughly twice as many men as women in Scotland have died because of alcohol (GRO Scotland, 2011). Men's high levels of drinking mean that the health benefits of lower consumption have not yet resulted in lower death rates (ONS, 2013b: 6). However, with binge drinking more common amongst young men it is not clear whether that improvement will come about. There is debate about whether young women are catching up, reflecting new feminine norms (Hunt and Batty, 2009).

Both gender and class are also implicated in smoking rates, the greatest single cause of premature death. In Britain smoking began as an 'elite' habit which then caught on amongst middle- and working-class men. Prior to the mid-1920s the main smokers were men. The tobacco industry, however, successfully promoted smoking differently for men and women, as a sign of masculinity for men, but also, especially after the Second World War, as the mark of a sophisticated and emancipated woman. This ensured that even when men began to smoke less in the 1960s due to health concerns, women's rates continued to increase. Today, rates of smoking are falling amongst both men and women and the percentage of women and men who smoke is almost the same (22% of men and 20% of women in 2009) (ONS, 2011b). Ideas about femininity and masculinity, however, are still important in understanding why people continue to smoke, especially people from disadvantaged backgrounds (Hunt et al., 2004).

The examples of smoking and drinking demonstrate that male and female bodies do not exist separately from the social context in which we live. For example, whilst oestrogen might protect women from CHD before menopause, smoking will nullify that protection (Annandale and Field, 2007: 95). Women's biological susceptibility to HIV is exacerbated by our lower social autonomy (Afifi, 2007: 385). Evidence suggests that women may be biologically more vulnerable to alcohol due to our different body mass and a difference in how we metabolize alcohol (Annandale, 2009) but whether women drink, how much, when and why is to not to do with our biology but to do with what is normal in society.

Implications for Practice

Gender inequality continues to be a feature of our health care system. Associated with this lack of gender equality is a lack of gender sensitivity. A traditional biomedical approach to health tends not to 'see' gender, preferring to view gendered behaviour as biological, rather than social. The danger of this approach is that it reinforces stereotypical views about men and women that are bad for our health. A woman who seems emotionally vulnerable or lacking in self-confidence about her treatment plan, for example, might not receive the support she needs because of a perception that this is just the way that women are. Alternatively, a man's insistence that he feels 'fine' might be accepted when it should not be. As the next chapter will show, gender stereotyping can also be particularly detrimental for lesbian, gay, bisexual and transgender people. The Equality Act (2010) requires public bodies like the NHS to monitor gender equality and take steps to redress inequalities, but health professionals themselves have a role to play in creating gender equality and sensitivity in their organizations. On an everyday level, this means learning to recognize gender issues. It means developing a capacity to tailor treatment to take account of the impact of masculinities and femininities on how individuals experience and understand their health problems (Annandale and Riska, 2009).

Summary

- To understand gendered health patterns it is necessary to consider the complex interaction of biological and social factors
- Gender inequality disadvantages women in particular ways, endangering their health
- Hegemonic masculinity also presents dangers for men's health which are social, not biological

Exercise

Ask three people (preferably not classmates) to answer these questions:

1. How many times have you been to see a doctor in the past year?
2. What is your gender?
3. What is your age group? (choose from: 0–15, 16–25, 26–45, 46–64, 65–79, 80+)

Compare your answers with other students. Try to explain your findings. Did you find a difference between men and women? What difference did age make? Are your results consistent with the data presented in this chapter?

Further Reading

Kuhlmann, E. and Annandale, E. (2012) *The Palgrave Handbook of Gender and Healthcare*. Second edition. Basingstoke: Palgrave Macmillan.
Payne, S. (2006) *The Health of Men and Women*. Cambridge: Polity.
Robertson, S. (2007) *Understanding Men and Health: Masculinities, Identity and Wellbeing*. Maidenhead: McGraw Hill, Open University Press.

Online readings

To access further resources related to this chapter, visit the companion website at www.sagepub.co.uk/russell

Springer, K. W. and Mouzon, D. M. (2011) '"Macho men" and preventative healthcare: Implications for older men in different social classes', *Journal of Health and Social Behavior*, 52(2): 212–27.

7

Sexuality

Key issues

- It is society, not biology, that shapes our sexual feelings and self-understanding
- Promoting sexual health means supporting people to express and enjoy their sexuality free of coercion, discrimination and violence
- Stigma and secrecy about unconventional sexual behaviour is a major threat to sexual health

---

Introduction

Images of sexuality are all around us in the media and wider society. Even if we are not having sex, it is part of our everyday lives. Yet sexuality means different things to different people. For some of us, it is an important part of our **identity**, an aspect of who we are. For most of us, sexuality is tied up with our hopes and dreams for a happy life and can bring pleasure, fun and intimacy. Yet it can also mean anxiety, discomfort, pain and even death. Some religious perspectives also view certain sexual behaviour as immoral and wrong. Not surprisingly, then, sexuality is a subject about which people feel emotional and hold strong opinions. From the perspective of health care, an unofficial working definition suggested by the World Health

Organization suggests seeing sexual health as 'a state of physical, emotional, mental and social well-being related to sexuality' involving 'pleasurable and safe sexual experiences, free of coercion, discrimination and violence' (World Health Organization, 2006). Despite much greater interest in recent years, of all the inequalities discussed in this book, sexual inequalities have received least attention and are most in need of enthusiastic advocacy within health and social care (Fish, 2010: 333; Gott et al., 2004). This chapter explores the **social construction** of our sexuality and what it means for our health.

A Short History of Sexuality

All societies have formal and informal rules and standards about the expression of sexuality and its consequences, rules about what we can do and with whom. These issues are inevitably connected to social **norms** about **gender**. 'Common sense' views about what is normal **masculinity and femininity** also involve ideas about who we should 'naturally' feel attracted to. Many studies from various societies confirm that both gender and sexuality have been expressed in a variety of ways. To give just one example, amongst the 'Sambia' of Papua New Guinea, a teenage boy becomes sexually mature by participating in a private ritual in which an older male acquaintance shows him how to perform oral sex. It is believed that by drinking the older man's semen, the boy acquires male strength. This ritual is not seen as 'gay'. It is just one stop on the road to adult sexuality in which boys will only have sex with women (Herdt, 2004).

This example is provocative because it challenges two 'common sense' ideas in our society about 'normal' sexuality. One of these, the idea that we should not have sex with people of the same gender as us, is a taboo which is no longer recognized as humane in most parts of the world. The other is a more deep-seated rule, which remains dominant worldwide: that adults should not be sexual with children. However, even this strong taboo is not universal historically. Relationships between men and boys were socially acceptable and common in ancient Greece and Rome, for example. Boys became sexually unattractive to men when they began to develop facial and pubic hair. These relationships were not 'gay' as men slept with both boys and women.

In other ways, the ancients laid the basis for attitudes to sexuality that persist in our society today, for example, in their admiration for 'self-control'. Whilst the Greeks and Romans were more concerned with resisting food than sex, the idea that the virtuous should turn their back on sensual pleasures survived into the Christian era, and sex became its main target. The early Christians saw sex as binding all people to the physical world and distancing them from heaven. Later Christians revised this view so that at least within marriage, sex was seen as acceptable and even positive. At the same time, they condemned any sexual practices that did not produce babies, including masturbation, anal and oral sex, sex between two men or two women and sex with animals, as well as attempts to avoid pregnancy in marriage (Mottier, 2008: 18–24).

However, the nineteenth-century rise of science saw the rules of proper sexual behaviour re-worked to fit this new world view. **Biomedicine** took conventional views about what was sexually normal and medicalized them. In particular, in 1868 a Hungarian journalist coined the term 'homosexual' (Takács, 2004). Whilst anal sex ('sodomy') had been forbidden for centuries, the invention of the 'homosexual' represented a new way of thinking about the act of anal sex between men. Basing itself in biomedicine, this new category cast a man who commits sodomy with another man as someone who does so habitually and prefers sex with men to any other kind. A person who committed this act was now a 'type' of person. It was an idea easily extended to women. The term 'lesbianism' appeared almost simultaneously in 1870 (Mottier, 2008: 38).

The birth of 'homosexuality' was not just about new rules about the sex of those we could be sexual with. It was also associated with the rise of a new social order which sought to control the genetic purity of nations (see also Chapter 4). 'Healthy' living meant having monogamous sex with a genetically appropriate person in the context of marriage to make healthy babies (Foucault, 1978). Any other kind of sex was framed as illicit and stigmatized as perverted or dangerous. Illicit sex included masturbation, which was considered a waste of sexual energy and believed to cause the disease of 'masturbatory insanity'. Symptoms included stammering, baldness, blindness and skin diseases (Engelhardt, 1981).

Women's sexuality was particularly threatening as biomedicine cast women's sexuality as responsive to men. Cutting the clitoris as a 'cure' for unwomanly behaviour was a common practice across Europe, for example. The new science of 'sexology' that developed at the turn of the twentieth century explained sexual behaviour as the expression of inbuilt instinctive drives and, inspired by Darwin, sought the answers to human sexuality in the animal world. Sexologists identified a long catalogue of 'perversions' to help identify people whose natural urges had developed wrongly (Mottier, 2008).

Reformers like Sigmund Freud, however, also introduced a new idea: that sexuality should be seen as a natural force which, if repressed, could lead to mental ill health and danger for society.

In the years following the Second World War, sexuality became the focus of public anxieties about private morality. This was a particularly frightening time to be gay. In Britain, gay people unable to keep their sexuality a secret faced unemployment, arrest, imprisonment and murder. In the late 1960s and early 1970s many gay men were treated by psychiatrists with electric shock aversion therapy to try to retrain their attraction to men, whilst lesbians were given desensitization and assertiveness training (Rogers and Pilgrim, 2010: 85).

Yet the stifling morality of the 1950s and 1960s also sparked radical social movements, including the women's movement and the gay rights movement. These movements challenged the 'naturalness' of both gender and sexuality. In particular, they condemned the role played by the medical profession in the ongoing pathologizing of gay sexuality. This was symbolized in the continued listing of homosexuality in the *Diagnostic and Statistical Manual of Mental Disorders* (DSM), the official document used to diagnose mental illness. When psychiatrists finally 'demedicalized' homosexuality by removing it from the DSM in 1974 it represented a recognition of the power of psychiatry to do damage through labelling (you will read more about labelling in Chapter 8) (Conrad and Angell, 2004).

The idea that diverse expressions of sexuality should be enjoyed and celebrated now became more widely held. New British legislation in the twenty-first century finally made it illegal to discriminate against people at work because of their sexuality and offered some legal rights for gay relationships. However, as later sections will explore, there have been real limits to our sexual liberation. Whilst greater diversity of sexual lives has enhanced the lives of many, its promise has also provoked old fears and anxieties connected to sexual conduct. This contradiction remains an essential aspect of the social context of current efforts to promote sexual health. It is important, then, to explore the issue of what is, and is not, sexually 'natural'.

The Social Construction of Sexuality

For many people the idea that our sexual desires, behaviours and identity are fixed by biology seems self-evident and unquestionable. The suggestion that this aspect of our lives is cultural, a product of society, may seem to fly in the face of everything we know about ourselves. 'Common sense' says that human sexuality can be explained by sexual drives, hormones and bio-chemical reactions in the brain. According to this theory, the male sex drive is stronger. It urges men to have heterosexual sex, to have it as much as possible, and to have it with more than one woman in order to 'spread his seed' and ensure the success of his genes. The female sex drive, on the other hand, is driven by a biological urge to have and nurture babies. Female sexuality is therefore weaker and more passive (women enjoy sex but they need to be wooed) and women find it easier to restrict themselves to one partner only (Weeks, 2010).

One problem with these 'common sense' ideas is that there are no examples of sexual behaviour that they *don't* claim to explain. Counter-examples are just taken as evidence of biological abnormality: there is something 'wrong' with those of us who don't conform. Moreover, as suggested in the introduction to this chapter, human sexual behaviour shows huge variety and has a history. Historical evidence suggests that our experiences of sexual pleasure are highly contextual. What we con-sider sexual is specific to our society. The ancients, for example, liked to touch and caress one another but did not associate this kind of touching with sexuality in the way that we do (Mottier, 2008). In our own society, context is very important for whether we will feel desire. Nakedness, for example, in the 'wrong' context, brings not desire, but embarrassment (see Case Study: Gloves).

. . . .

Gloves

In a medical encounter, professional and patient are protected from discomfort by the use of objects which can be seen as props in a theatre aimed at de-sexualizing nakedness. A woman having a smear test, for example, will usually have a thin sheet placed over the lower half of her body, a demure layer between herself and the professional performing the procedure. Another useful prop is latex gloves. Gloves are important for protecting against infection and, as Julia Twigg suggests, for protecting health and social care workers from some of the 'less attractive' aspects of their work: 'it's nice not to get somebody's faeces under your fingernails'. However, gloves also have a particular social function. Twigg studied the ways that careworkers bathing service users used and talked about gloves. Her conclusion was that, in addition to their medical and hygiene func-tions, gloves provide a way for workers 'to protect themselves from the full

(Continued)

CASE STUDY

(Continued)

intimacy of bathing work', to 'put up a barrier of professionalism between the client and the worker' (404). In this quote, one of the careworkers she interviewed reflects on how gloves can symbolically protect workers from touch that is too direct and intimate:

> [...] I suppose, with men in particular, I think it's quite appreciated to wear, I appreciate wearing them [...] you know they might get into it having a nice girl rubbing their back with bare hands [...] Having the gloves, it's kind of like wearing a badge saying: I am here for a reason, this is what I'm doing. I'm not just here with you naked, washing you [...] I felt better about it.

Source: Twigg, J. (2000) 'Carework as a form of bodywork', *Ageing and Society*, 20: 389–411.

Whilst there may be clear biological parameters to sexual experience, how we experience sexual pleasure is not fixed by biology but enacted within a culture. Television, books, playground chatter, our parents and the internet all provide a repertoire of possible ways that sexuality can be understood and experienced. In this, our rules about sex are similar to our rules about dressing, table manners and eating (Weeks, 2010). There are some things, for example, which no human being will enjoy eating, such as rotting food. However, international cuisine suggests that within such restrictions there is great diversity in terms of what we can learn to enjoy eating, and some capacity for development and change, even when we are adults. When it comes to enjoying sex, as with food, social structures constrain the range of possibilities that lie before us. Those possibilities are not just part of the social world outside us but the social world as it comes to exist within us (Parker, 2009).

One way the social world exists within us is in the way we come to understand our sexual identity. When we think about who we want to be with, we do so with reference to categories of sexual identity supplied to us by our society. In particular, sexual identities reflect the way in which sexuality in our society has been medicalized. The idea that some people are biologically wired to be attracted to one sex throughout their life continues to be influential. Even today the idea that some people have sex with men because they have a 'gay gene' or a 'gay brain' has received surprising support given how little evidence exists in support of it

(O'Riordan, 2012). Part of the popularity of this idea is that it might seem to offer support for gay people – they were just 'born that way'. For some, who have found being gay in this society profoundly traumatic, it offers the possibility of treatment and a 'cure'.

However, a fundamental problem for attempts to identify any biological characteristic shared by gay people is establishing who is and is not 'homosexual'. A number of studies now confirm evidence first compiled in 1948 that large numbers of men have sex with other men but see themselves as heterosexual. A 1970 study found that the majority of men meeting in public toilets for casual sex considered themselves heterosexual and many were happily married. A substantial minority of people who identify as gay men continue to have occasional sex with women. It is also common for people, especially women, to change their sexual identity over the course of their lives. They might, for example, grow up 'heterosexual', have a husband and children and then live the rest of their life as a lesbian, or the other way round (Wilton, 2000). For this reason, some research into sexual health, particularly Sexually Transmitted Diseases (STDs), now uses categories like 'Men Who Have Sex with Men' (MSMs) and 'Men Who Only Have Sex with Women' (MSWs) to focus on behaviour rather than identity (Marongiu et al., 2012). The search for a gay 'gene' or brain, therefore, is misguided. In a society in which identifying yourself as 'gay' is likely to have at least some negative consequences, how people define themselves will not necessarily accord with what they do. The following section outlines some of the negative health consequences of same sex attraction that lead many people to choose to keep their same sex attractions a secret.

Health Patterns of LGBT People in Britain

Lesbian, gay, bisexual and **transgender** (LGBT) people comprise 6% of the UK population (Fish, 2010). 'Transgender' refers to anyone who does not easily fit into the social norm of two mutually exclusive and biologically defined sexes with ascribed roles and behaviours. This may be because of how they express their gender or identify themselves or because they are intersex, having been born or developing physical features that might fit with being male or female (Agius and Tobler, 2012: 12). Whilst the health problems of LGBT people have only recently begun to be routinely surveyed (Edwards, 2012), it is difficult to see any impact of the improved status of LGBT people in society in recent decades when we consider health statistics. LGBT people have worse mental health than the general population. This is especially true for transgender and bisexual people. Gay and bisexual men are four times more likely to commit suicide and LBT women are also much more likely than others to commit suicide. Transgender people are particular at risk to being victims of violence, substance abuse and suicide. LGBT people have a higher rate of alcohol consumption and of difficulties related to alcohol. Lesbians and bisexual women are particularly likely to misuse substances and bisexual men are more likely than both gay and heterosexual men to use recreational drugs (Barker et al., 2012; Edwards, 2012; Fish, 2010; King et al., 2008; McAndrew and Warne, 2004).

Given their higher risk of mental ill health, it is not surprising that LGBT people also have higher rates of physical ill health. Self-reported health status is worse for LBT women than other women. LGBT people more frequently report acute physical symptoms and chronic conditions. Because LGBT people are more likely to smoke they are at greater risk for lung cancer. Lesbian and bisexual women may also be more likely to develop breast cancer because they are less likely to have children (childbirth is protective against breast cancer). Whilst rates of HIV/AIDS amongst GBT men had been declining, many countries now report an increased prevalence. GBT men are also at higher risk of hepatitis B and C. However, whilst bisexual people have been mistakenly blamed by some for transmitting HIV and other STDs into heterosexual and lesbian communities, statistics suggest that bisexual men have lower rates of HIV infection than gay men (Barker et al., 2012; Addis et al., 2009; Edwards, 2012, Fish, 2010).

These patterns reflect the everyday stigma, discrimination and resultant psychosocial stress which LGBT people experience. Unfortunately, many experiences of discrimination occur in health care settings. In Britain until 2004 it was not illegal for care workers to deny access to care to partners of same-sex patients and exclude them from decision-making. Fish and Hunt (2008) report that only 30% of the women they spoke to felt that the practitioner refrained from making inappropriate comments and only 10% felt that their partner was really included in the consultation process. Transgender people in particular report high levels of insensitive and disrespectful attitudes and behaviour. A 2003 UK study found one third of bisexual men reported that health professionals had made a link between their sexuality and a mental health problem (cited in Barker et al., 2012: 27)(Edwards, 2012; Fish, 2010; Royal College of Nursing, 2005). Other problems arise from a lack of knowledge by professionals about LGBT health. Lesbian and bisexual women are advised by some GPs that they are not at risk for cervical cancer and therefore not eligible for screening as they do not have sex with men. Yet 19% of women who have never had sex with a man have the Human Papillomavirus (HPV) virus which can lead to cervical cancer (Fish, 2010; Fish and Hunt, 2008).

Not surprisingly, as a consequence, many, if not, most LGBT people keep their sexuality a secret from their GP and other health care professionals. A 2008 UK study found half of LBT women had not told their GP of their sexuality. Levels of disclosure are also very low among transgender and **intersex** people. This explains why GPs and other health service providers often believe, in error, that they have no LGBT patients. When Sally Knocker contacted care homes to conduct research with older gay and lesbian people she was commonly told 'You won't find anyone gay here' (Knocker, 2012: 13). One consequence is that LGBT people fail to engage with health services, for fear of experiencing disrespect (Barker et al., 2012; Edwards, 2012, Fish and Hunt, 2008) (see Case Study: 'My Biggest Fear').

....

'My Biggest Fear'

A study of lesbian, gay and bisexual people aged over 55 in England, Scotland and Wales by Stonewall in 2010 revealed their anxieties about their treatment by health and social care workers. One in six lesbian and bisexual women and one in nine gay and bisexual men had experienced discrimination, hostility or poor treatment when using GP services because of their sexual orientation.

> 'Although things are improving, there is still a lot of ignorance at least, homophobia at worst, among health and social care people' (Rita, 61, South East).

> 'I have had bad experiences with social services and carers, in respect that I was cautioned not to mention I am gay, in case a carer did not approve' (Harry, 74, London).

> 'I am a gay woman in a very loving and long relationship... My biggest fear is that if we both become ill and need care that we might be separated or be looked after by people who are anti-gay and would treat us badly' (Sheila, 62, North West).

> 'Moving to the West Midlands five years ago from the South East I have been shocked by the unfriendliness and lack of understanding of the staff in my GP surgery' (Martin, 62, West Midlands).

(Continued)

CASE STUDY

(Continued)

> 'I do not want to be looked after by someone who dislikes me because I am a lesbian' (Shaila, 57, South East)

> 'The thought of being in my own home requiring help and someone who brings in with them the prejudices and judgements of the world I experience "out there" fills me with dread' (James, 55, London).

Source: Guasp, A. (2011) *Lesbian, Gay and Bisexual People in Later Life*. London: Stonewall. See also: Heaphy, B. (2009) 'The storied, complex lives of older LGBT adults', *Journal of GLBT Family Studies*, 5: 119–38.

Social Factors in Sexual Health: Heterosexism

Why does this discrimination continue, despite legislation introduced to counter it? One answer is that some health care professionals believe homosexuality is immoral, for religious reasons. However, those who make this judgement are misreading religious texts, such as the Bible or the Koran, as homosexuality did not exist before the 1890s. New laws reject the claim that disapproving of homosexuality is a private matter and defend the rights of sexual minorities to respectful care. For example, if there is a conflict between a GP's own moral belief and the patient's treatment, the GP must explain this and give the patient the right to see another GP (General Medical Council, 2006, cited in Fish, 2010: 336).

However, evidence suggests that disrespect is not always deliberate. Sexuality may be a confronting issue for health and social care practitioners (Haboubi and Lincoln, 2003). Many of the injuries caused to LGBT people are a consequence of assuming that people are heterosexual (Fish, 2010: 335). A useful way to understand these problems is to see them as reflecting **heterosexism** in society. Chapters 4, 5 and 6 in this book explored ways in which **racism, ageism** and sexism result in health disadvantages for ethnic minority and older people and women. It is helpful to also recognize our society as heterosexist. Julie Fish defines heterosexism as:

> ...a belief system which values heterosexuality as superior to homosexuality, assumes that everyone is, or should be, heterosexual, and intersects with other forms of oppression such as racism and sexism (2010: 337).

The heterosexual 'norm' influences 'the status people are accorded, the power they can exercise and the life-chances open to them' (Edwards, 2012: 292, citing Lorber and Moore, 2002). For example, sexuality and gender work together to create hierarchies in which some groups are visible and legitimate and others, less so. Our place in this hierarchy has implications for our health status (Corr et al., 2008). For example, the high rates of mental health problems of bisexual people are directly related to the low status of bisexual people in terms of both legitimacy and visibility (Barker et al., 2012: 4).

Social Factors: Stigma

One way that heterosexism disadvantages LGBT people is through stigma. The sociologist Erving Goffman, in his 1963 book *Stigma*, noted two kinds of outsiders in society. The first were 'deviants', those who had broken social rules. The second were people who had broken no rule but simply because of who they were had come to be identified as in some way 'spoiled' and shameful. In recent decades many observers have recognized stigma as a barrier to health care (Scambler, 2008: 215). It has been particularly damaging in relation to HIV/AIDS. Constructive efforts to halt the spread of the disease have, since its emergence in 1981, been thwarted by a focus on

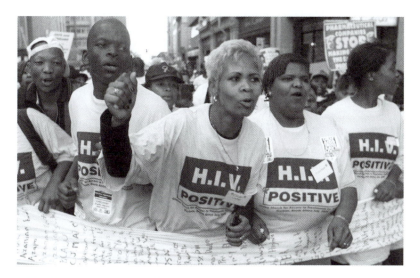

Figure 7.1   Rejecting stigma. Demonstrators march in Durban, 9 July 2000, on the first day of the XIII International AIDS Conference

Photograph courtesy Corbis Images

blaming various groups who have caught the disease, including gay men, intravenous drug users and black Africans. The example of HIV/AIDS also demonstrates how stigma links to social structure (see Figure 7.1). Stigma is usually associated, for example, with other forms of disadvantage and political powerlessness (Link and Phelan, 2001; Deacon and Stephney, 2007, Poundstone et al., 2004; Scambler, 2009) (see Case Study: Social Factors in the Spread of HIV).

CASE STUDY

Social Factors in the Spread of HIV

Sanyu Mojola (2011) links the HIV epidemic in sub-Saharan Africa to the 'eco-social' environment. Damage caused by deforestation to Lake Victoria, Africa's largest freshwater lake (and a major site for the epidemic), changed relationships between people in ways that increased their HIV risk. The deteriorating quality of the lake has meant that local fisherman spend more time away from home seeking fertile fishing grounds. This has meant they are more likely to have sex with different people at different sites. In addition, fishing, as in other parts of the world, is a dangerous occupation for men whose masculinity is tied up risking their lives due to drowning or fatal encounters with hippos, crocodiles and pirates. Whilst many lakeside residents spend weekends attending or planning funerals, fishermen continue to resist using condoms, despite education campaigns, because of this masculine identity and their perception that wearing condoms reduces the pleasure of sex. The economic dependence of local women on the fishermen in turn makes it difficult for them to demand safe sex or monogamous relationships. Mojola argues that her account demonstrates that encouraging people to change their individual behaviour without recognizing and addressing the circumstances in which they are making those choices may fail.

Source: Mojola, S.A. (2011) 'Fishing in dangerous waters: Ecology, gender and economy in HIV risk', *Social Science and Medicine*, 72(2) January 2011: 149–56.

Celebrating Sexuality?

Whilst stigma can be seen as one aspect of powerlessness, it should be noted that episodes from the history of LGBT activism also highlight that people on the receiving end of stigma do not passively internalize negative images of themselves. Many who have been targets of stigma, included those considered disabled, mentally ill and 'perverted', have taken the negative 'spoiled' identities that have been foisted on them and remade them in their own image. They have made them a basis for solidarity, pride and celebration instead of atomization, shame and blame (Scambler and Paoli, 2008). 'Coming out', for example, has been used by gay people as a powerful narrative of resistance to stigma (Ridge and Ziebland, 2012).

From this perspective, LGBT people can be seen as being in the frontline of sexual health, their experiences and struggles against stigma relevant to the sexual health of all. With sexuality an arena in which people are increasingly willing to express their individuality, sexual lives have become more diverse. The internet has provided a safe place for people to experiment with new sexual behaviours, for example through the use of avatars (see Figure 7.2). Yet most scientists in the field of sexuality remain firmly resistant to explaining these changes by reference to social factors, preferring to identify new sexual lifestyles as variations of 'pathology' (Cacchioni and Tiefer, 2012). **Medicalization** continues to frame sexuality in general, not only in relation to LGBT people.

For example, not enjoying or being able to have sex has been increasingly constructed as a medical problem which can be treated biochemically (see Case Study in Chapter 2: Orgasm Inc). Women's moods and ageing are framed as hormonal problems, leading to the idea that problems of men as they age may also be understood as a kind of menopause. Poor body image has been conceptualized as a medical problem which must be treated surgically. For transgender people this has been a human rights issue. Availability of surgery for this group is about their right to alter their

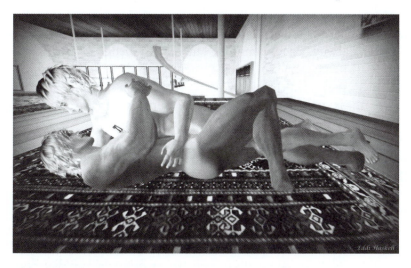

Figure 7.2 Virtual sex: avatars

From www.eddihaskell.com, image courtesy Eddi Haskell

external appearance to fit their inner identity. More generally, recent years have seen a growing emphasis, even pressure, to view enthusiasm for sex as a sign and symbol of good health (Marshall, 2012).

Yet whilst some of us are pathologized because of how we express our sexuality, the association of sexuality with fertility and hence with youth, good health and an 'able' body has meant that some people are expected not to be sexual at all. Some disabled people have been forced to lobby in order to draw attention to their sexual needs in care settings, struggling against a perception that they are asexual (Milligan and Neufeldt, 2001). Similarly, the assumption by health care professionals that older people will be or should be asexual has resulted in inadequate care (Heath, 2002). The sexuality of dying people has been described as one of health care's last taboos, though research shows that sex remains important to many people even as they are dying (Cort et al., 2004; Wells, 2002; Searle, 2002; Smolinksi and Colón, 2011).

Implications for Practice

Discussions about sexuality in relation to health have tended to reinforce two stereotypical images. On the one hand, the loving, monogamous heterosexual couple whose 'sex life' is interrupted by ill health or fatigue (and can be 'saved' by Viagra or other drugs). On the other, the promiscuous sexual deviants whose irresponsible lust spreads HIV and other STDs. The reality is that most people's lives do not conform to either of these stereotypes. Most gay families are loving and monogamous and there are many heterosexual people who have had more than one sexual partner and may have failed to always use a condom. The real challenge for sexual health is not 'immoral' behaviour but social structures and policies which promote stigma and secrecy. Health care workers in all professionals, not just those who work in sexual health, need to develop awareness about sexuality issues that may affect health as part of gender awareness.

Summary

- Sexual health involves social, not just biological factors
- Sexual inequality has resulted in patterns of poor health for people who are not heterosexual
- Promoting good sexual health means being aware of and countering the implications of heterosexism and stigma

Exercise

1. List characteristics you would associate with a sexually healthy person.
2. Sexuality is an emotional issue. This can make it challenging to think about. Did this chapter push you out of your comfort zone? What kind of issues might arise in your professional practice that might challenge you in this way? Discuss and explore.

Further Reading

Fish, J. (2006) *Heterosexism in Health and Social Care*. Basingstoke, UK: Palgrave.

Wilton, T. (2000) *Sexualities in Health and Social Care*. Buckingham, Philadelphia: Open University Press. Whilst this book is a little dated, it nonetheless provides an excellent introduction.

8

Chronic illness and disability

Key issues

- Experiences of chronic illness and disability reflect the social context in which symptoms and impairments occur
- Discrimination is a major social factor impacting on the health of disabled people and those with chronic illness
- How biomedical knowledge is shared is important for the management of chronic illness and disability

Introduction

Illness is often spoken about as if it is something that happens to us from time to time, but then, we get better and our bodies return to 'normal'. For those of us who have chronic illness or a disability, this way of thinking is problematic. It reflects a biomedical framework for thinking about health and illness. As suggested in Chapter 1, the biomedical model of health, whilst it is based on science and offered an improved approach to health, suffered from certain inadequacies. It tended to reduce bodies to machines and to disregard the thinking and emotional aspects of people as well as the wider social circumstances in which they live. The tension between the benefits of medical science and the limitations of an approach that tends to reduce people to their bodies is felt especially keenly in the lives of people who have chronic illness and disability. This chapter explores the importance of social factors in shaping the experiences of people in these categories.

A Short History of Chronic Illness and Disability

For most people today and in previous societies, hard lives and exposure to germs or violence commonly resulted in death at a young age. The experience of having a medical condition which lasts over months and years has been exceptional historically. Until recently, most human bodies did not last long enough to become 'old' and in the majority world this is still the case for many people. For those who did live for many years with physical characteristics that were different from others, life depended on how that difference was understood, which always reflected the wider ideas of the time. In ancient society, for example, the birth of a child with a twisted limb would be understood as a negative sign from the Gods, a portent. The child might be killed or expelled from society. They might be forced to support themselves by begging and be openly derided (Garland, 1995: 44, cited in Barnes and Mercer, 2010: 15).

Yet some records also suggest that those who were disabled or ill were treated and taken care of. The association of people we would now see as disabled with the supernatural even meant they might also be seen as having special abilities (Stiker, 2000). For centuries, this basic frame stayed in place. Disabled people were considered to be sinners at heart, their physical state a punishment from God. However, alongside this, religious traditions encouraged charity towards such sinners.

In mid-nineteenth century Britain, reforms of the Poor Laws (discussed in Chapter 5) established more firmly that people with physical or mental impairments were, like the old, unlucky rather than bad, and therefore deserving of charity. These laws marked a change that would become worldwide. This did not mean that life was necessarily better for disabled people after that time. Agricultural regimes had a flexibility which meant that family members with physical vulnerabilities could be incorporated in production in a way that they could not in a factory.

There were also some other changes in society, much more subtle, but nonetheless important, which added to the disadvantage of some disabled people. We take it for granted today that substances which routinely come out of our bodies are distasteful and should be disposed of discretely. We go to the toilet in private, avoid farting in public, blow snot into a tissue and hold our mouth closed when we chew. Yet it has not always been so. Most people throughout history were not trained to control their bodies in this way nor to be disgusted by those who did not. It was only in the eighteenth century, starting in the courts of wealthy elites, that this kind of body control came to be admired and then emulated throughout society (Elias, 2000). One indirect consequence of this new focus on bodily restraint was that people with weaker organs and less ability to achieve this control were now at an added disadvantage.

Thanks to **biomedicine,** many people (albeit mostly in the wealthiest countries) have lived who would have died. Some painful conditions have been cured or made less painful, though not evenly throughout the world. In addition, the idea of the mind/body distinction (see Chapter 1), at least in theory, suggested that disabled and chronically ill people could demand to be treated as human beings worthy of equality, despite their physical differences. Whilst previous societies tended to see personal qualities as fixed by God, **the Enlightenment** brought enthusiasm for the idea that all people could 'improve' themselves. However, there were also extremely negative aspects to biomedicine. In the same way that gerontology turned old age into a disease and gave it a biomedical inevitability it had not had previously, biomedicine created categories for people whose minds and bodies did not function like most others.

Being slotted into many of these categories could have dire consequences for individuals. The nineteenth century saw the rise of 'total institutions' including prisons, workhouses and asylums. These were places for those displaced by the rise of industrialism, unable to conform to clock-watching or the faster pace of factory production. For disabled people, total institutions were presented as an environment in which they could become better people but within a wider social frame which portrayed them as objects of pity whose physical bodies imposed strict and wide-reaching limitations on the kinds of lives they might possibly be able to enjoy.

One particularly negative intellectual trend for disabled people which arose in the 1890s was the **eugenics movement** (introduced in Chapter 4). Eugenicists, influential across the world, viewed physical, learning and emotional disabilities as symptoms of poor genes, of bad breeding. In the early twentieth century, scientists influenced by eugenics devised schemas classifying human beings according to their supposed intelligence and proscribing the **social class** locations felt appropriate for each level of development. Tens of thousands of Americans were sterilized in the early twentieth century under government policies inspired by eugenics (Bruinius, 2007).

The idea that people with impairments are genetically inferior represented a low point in humanity's characterization of disability, which culminated in the murder of many thousands of disabled people in the Holocaust. Nazi ideology, following eugenics, argued that disabled people, along with Black and Jewish people and criminals, were the result of 'poor breeding' and society would be best served by removing them from the so-called 'gene pool' (Brown and Brown, 2003). It was only after the Second World War that a more humane global environment resulted in reforms such as the British 1948 National Assistance Act. This Act defined 'disability', set out what percentage of 'abnormality' or 'loss' was associated with particular conditions and made economic provision for disabled people (Barnes and Mercer, 2010: 17–19).

Increasingly, disabled people were moved out of asylums, hospitals and other institutions with sociologists such as Erving Goffman drawing attention to the ways in which 'total institutions' imposed a distorted identity on those living there (Goffman, 1961). By the 1970s, being 'provided for' no longer represented the extent of the aspirations and expectations of disabled people. They began to organize a movement aimed at fundamentally changing the way disabled people were viewed and treated.

Chronic Illness and Disability in the UK

In 2009 around 30% of adults in Britain reported that they had a long-standing illness or disability, increased from 21% in 1972 (ONS, 2011b: 3). The terms 'chronic illness' and 'disability' do not mean the same thing. A person who has a disability may not in any sense be ill. For example, their impairment may be the result of a single event in the past or a congenital condition (3% of disabled people have had their condition since birth) (Williams et al., 2008: 7). At the same time, a person who has a chronic illness may be prevented by bodily symptoms from doing very much at all on one day but not the next, and so their degree of impairment is not fixed.

However, there are many overlaps between the two categories. As argued in Chapter 1, our ideas of what it means to be 'ill' are socially constructed and the same is true of the idea of 'disability', as will be explored in more detail later in this chapter. For example, changes to the

2005 Disability Discrimination Act expanded the definition of disability to include people who have impairments as a result of having had the diseases cancer, multiple sclerosis and HIV (15% of disabled people fall into this category)(Williams et al., 2008: 7).

What is certainly true is that long-term physical conditions, whether constantly debilitating or virtually trivial, are being experienced by a growing proportion of people in society. In many countries, infectious disease continues to be the main health issue. In wealthier countries like Britain, however, chronic disease has overtaken infectious disease as living standards have improved. Today, health care professionals in Britain spend much more time 'caring' for people who have a long-term condition than they do trying to 'cure' people with acute conditions. Such conditions range from those which are very painful much or even all of the time (arthritis, fibromyalgia, back problems) to those which are intermittently painful (sickle cell disease and thalassaemia) to those which are never painful (such as congenital blindness). Some chronic illnesses are not painful but can involve episodes which are highly distressing (asthma, epilepsy and stroke).

With a growing proportion of older people in society (and medicine's success in keeping some people alive who might previously have died), the importance of chronic conditions will only increase. Though many chronic illnesses and disabilities occur at all ages, people are more likely to suffer from a chronic illness or disability as they get older and there are particular disorders which are overwhelmingly experienced by older people such as arthritis, dementia, Parkinson's disease and stroke. In 2009, for example, 66% of people aged 75 suffered from a long-standing illness (ONS, 2011b: 3).

In relation to disability, the most commonly reported impairments affect mobility, lifting or carrying; others involve vision, hearing and learning. However, the chance of having an impairment increases with age so that whilst 6% of children are disabled, this rises to 15% of those of working age and 45% of those over State Pension age in the UK (ONS, 2010/11). Whilst about half of disabled people acquired their impairment, condition or disability before they were 50, about one-third have more than one impairment, with the number of impairments increasing with age (Williams et al., 2008: 7).

In addition, about 1.5 million people in the UK – 3% – have a learning disability. Learning disabilities are acquired before, during or after birth and affect ability to learn, communicate and do everyday things such as getting dressed, cooking or holding a conversation. Those with a severe learning disability, a minority, may require 24-hour care. People with a learning disability have a shorter life expectancy and increased risk of early death, though for some groups life expectancy is increasing. Those with moderate to severe learning disabilities have mortality rates three times higher than in the general popula-tion. Relatively common but potentially preventable causes of death include aspirational pneumonia and seizures (Emerson et al., 2012: 2). One important issue for health care professionals working with people with learning disabili-ties is how end-of-life decisions should be made (Wagemans et al., 2010).

The Medical and Social Models of Disability

The starting place for understanding both chronic illness and disability in the UK is the disability movement's critique of the biomedical model. There are a number of particular problems with the biomedical model for chroni-cally ill and disabled people. In Chapter 1 it was argued that biomedicine, by focusing on the biological aspects of our existence, neglects the psycho-logical and social. Its focus on the individual makes health our own busi-ness, which means that wider social forces and patterns which produce ill health, such as poverty, are background issues for biomedicine. For disabled people this focus on the individual and what can be done about their phys-ical state is particularly problematic. Biomedicine approaches diagnosis by comparing a person's bodily symptoms to what is 'normal', that is, most statistically common, and then trying to change the body and/or to make them more 'normal'. If something about your body is a problem for you, biomedicine may offer a way to reduce or remove that problem. The job of health care professionals is then to restore the body, as if it were a machine, to its normal functioning.

The lives of disabled people have been improved by these kinds of inter-ventions. Biomedical interventions such as pain relief, hip replacements, prostheses, wheelchairs and other aids for living can make life very much better. The problem is the biomedical idea of what is 'normal' is not sim-ply an objective, scientific standpoint but reflects social ideas about how bodies should look and function. If the angle of a person's limb is causing them pain, there may be little argument between them and their GP about the need for biomedical intervention to change that angle to reduce the pain. In other instances, however, the biomedical presumption of a need to 'correct' may be extremely problematic for a disabled person. For example, for some disabled people, there may be one part of their body that does not function in the same way that it does for most other people. However, this 'impairment' may not in itself pose any problem for that person. It may not cause them pain or inconvenience. It may be that the only negatives associated with this physical difference are associated, not with the body itself, but with other people who don't understand the nature and impact of that impairment.

For example, the invention of cochlear implants, electronic devices that can provide a sense of sound to people with hearing impairments, was viewed by the biomedical community as the breakthrough ('miracle cure') that would change the lives of hearing impaired people. This was not the reaction of many in the Deaf community and Deaf studies scholars. They rejected the idea of deafness as a disability, seeing it rather as the basis of a shared identity, culture and language (sign language). From this view, Deaf people are a linguistic minority and cochlear implants do not 'cure' a Deaf person but place them in a world without identity – neither Deaf nor hearing (Blume, 2010). The best thing for Deaf children, from this viewpoint, is to provide them with the cultural resources – sign language in particular – to enable them to participate in Deaf culture. The alternative is 'Oralism', education focused on speech and listening skills, which devalues Sign Language, and 'Audism', the devaluing of Deafness (Ladd, 2003).

For disability activists, the assumption that there is something wrong with their bodies – that they are 'abnormal' – is a reflection of a society dominated by people who do not have impairments. It is a society which does not make provision for people with impairments that creates disability, literally 'disabling' them. Whilst biomedicine constructs disability as a feature of individuals, disability activists have argued convincingly for a **social model of disability** which understands disability as a product of a particular kind of society. As the following sections will explore, disability is created by material factors such as employment and transport which go hand in hand with cultural factors such as stigma and discrimination. Disablement, Michael Oliver famously wrote 'is nothing to do with the body. It is a consequence of social oppression' (Oliver, 1996: 35).

Social model of disability: emphasizes that disability occurs when society fails to take the necessary steps to facilitate full participation of people who have impairments.

The implications of the disability movement's challenge are profound for those involved in health and social care. Concepts like 'rehabilitation' and even 'care', itself, have been criticized as disabling:

Rehabilitation can be seen as a major instrument of bodily rationalisation. Disguised as 'scientific' and operating under the banner of biomedicine, reha-bilitation is a powerful agent in the ratification of particular types of bodies... Common to most rehabilitation work, however, is a set of moral ideas about what bodies should be like (Seymour, 1998: 20, cited in Earle, 2003: 8).

For people with chronic illness, the individualist focus of biomedicine is also a problem. Refusing to engage with the medical establishment is usually not an option for someone managing a long-term condition. Science offers the possibility of finding a cure or, if none can be found, the best way we have of reducing daily symptoms and suffering. However, chronic illness is not just about the body. It is about changes that affect a person's whole life: their work, their relationships with other people, their future and their sense of who they are. A traditional biomedical approach to illness has little to offer people trying to negotiate all these aspects of life and not just the bio-logical. The following sections will consider some of the social factors that frame the challenges faced by people with disabilities or chronic illness.

Disadvantage

As Chapter 3 suggested, being ill is a socio-economic disadvantage. Being chronically ill or disabled makes a major difference to a person's chance of being un- or under-employed and living in poverty. This relationship works both ways. Amongst those least advantaged in society there are much higher rates of chronic illness and disability. As long ago as the nineteenth century Friedrich Engels (see Chapter 3) noted the systematic ways in which hard work-ing lives damaged human bodies. He observed mill hands with malformed spines, metal and steel workers with 'hind-leg', grinders with lung disease, pot-ters with skin disease, arsenic poisoning and paralysis, glass workers with eye disease, bowel and 'rheumatic and bronchial affections' (Synnott, 1993: 252). Today, people from lower **socio-economic** strata are more likely to experience chronic illness and disability and more likely to experience financial, domestic and work-related difficulties as a result (Field and Kelly, 2007: 142).

In turn, for those who have a disability obtaining employment is a par-ticular concern. Forty-six per cent of disabled people in Britain of working age are in work compared with 76% of the general population. Having a mental health condition is an even greater disadvantage, with only 17% in paid work. Disabled people are also less likely to be in managerial or profes-sional occupations and more likely to be employed in 'elementary' occupa-tions (postal worker, bar staff, warehouse assistant) (ONS, 2012e). This has inevitable consequences for economic wellbeing. Twenty per cent of people in families with at least one disabled member live in relative poverty on a Before Housing Costs basis, compared to 15% of those in families with no disabled members (ONS, 2010/11).

A number of factors lie behind the poor employment situation of disabled people (half of those with impairments face at least one **barrier** to employment). For those who are unemployed, the most important of these is ill health, which was a barrier for 43% of adults with impairments in 2009–11. Other major barriers include lack of job opportunities, difficulty with transport, family responsibilities, lack of qualifications or experience and anxiety or lack of confidence. One of the most important enablers for disabled people is modified or reduced hours or days of work. Education is also a key area where disabled people face barriers (ONS, 2012f). One 2007 survey found that nearly half of disabled people felt there were barriers to using health services especially the journey itself due to transport difficulties, distances and needing someone to accompany them (Williams et al., 2008).

> Barrier: a physical, social or economic obstacle that prevents the equal participation of disabled people in society.

Particular groups of disabled people also face specific challenges. For example, families of people with learning disabilities are more likely to be poor or become poor. In 2003/4 nearly one third of 13–14-year-old adolescents with learning disabilities reported being bullied at least weekly. Only 17% of working age adults with learning disabilities have paid employment. In 2009/11 British adults with learning disabilities were nearly three times more likely to have been victims of violent crime over the last year and seven times more likely to have been a victim of disability **hate crime**. In addition, people with learning disabilities who show challenging behaviour are especially at risk of ill health (Emerson et al., 2012: 11, 20).

As these statistics show, the low incomes of disabled people are tied up with a variety of factors which work together to disadvantage them economically. Some of the factors which have received particular attention include stigma and loss of self. The following section explores these issues and some of the ways that our understanding of chronic illness and disability have evolved in recent years.

Hate crime: a criminal offence committed against a person or property motivated by hostility towards someone based on their disability, race, religion, gender identity or sexual orientation.

Factors in Disadvantage for Chronically Ill and Disabled People

Chapter 7 introduced the idea of stigma and how it can endanger sexual health. A great deal of research has explored the impact of stigma on disabled people, including the mentally ill (see Chapter 9). The most direct and shocking result of stigma towards disabled people is violence. This is particularly, but not only, a problem for disabled people living in institutions. Both children and adults with disabilities are at much higher risk of violence than those who are not disabled. Children with disabilities are 3.7 times more likely to experience violence, rising to 4.6 times for children with mental or intellectual impairments (Jones et al., 2012). Adults are 1.5 times more likely to experience violence, rising to nearly 4 times more likely if they have a mental health condition (Hughes et al., 2012). People with disabilities are also especially vulnerable to a distinctive form of hate crime known as 'mate crime', where they are subjected to acts of cruelty, humiliation, servitude, exploitation and theft by people who are close to them (Thomas, 2011).

As mentioned in Chapter 7, it was Erving Goffman who pioneered our understanding of stigma. Along with Irving Zola (see Chapter 2), Goffman was a radical who was critical of conventional society and sympathetic to those who broke social rules. In particular, these thinkers were interested in the damage done to individuals as a result of being diagnosed by medical gatekeepers as 'abnormal'. Goffman's writing had clear implications for disabled people. In his 1963 book *Asylums*, for example, he explored how psychiatric hospitals, prisons and monasteries force identity change on people who live there. Work, leisure, eating and sleeping are merged into a 'batch living' environment akin to a factory farm with the consequence that a process of 'mortification of self' occurs. Wearing a uniform helps this process along, one of a variety of 'degradation rituals' which work with strict routines and time discipline to reorganize the self and impose a devalued identity. Writing about *Stigma*, Goffman explored how being labelled as 'abnormal' and of less value than others can lead to discrimination and a feeling of being 'lesser' (see Case Study: Mabel Cooper and Figure 8.2).

Mabel Cooper

Mabel Cooper was a resident in St Lawrence's Hospital, a long-stay institution for people with learning disabilities. Dorothy Atkinson worked with her to publish the story of her life. In this extract, she looks back:

> For people like me, and a lot more, you know, people were frightened of us. So in them days they said OK, there's nowhere for you, you get shut away in the big institutions. If people are different then other people get frightened. I still see it. People are frightened of people like me, and a lot more, because we're different.
>
> I go into the schools now, and talk to the children, and I've been invited back to the schools, so for the next three weeks I'm off into the schools. But, you know, they were frightened, they even told me, the children. They're frightened of people that are different.
>
> I got into the system very early. It was only because I had the learning disability, they've found that out now. I was born at the wrong time. Because I always say to the children, if I was young again I would have liked to have gone to the school, and learnt all the things I don't know now. The only thing is, when you start going in places like that, they label you and that's it.
>
> St Lawrence's was all I knew for years, it was all I knew until 15 or 16 years ago. When you're in there you don't know anything else. There was nice people like Eva, she was nice. I got on with her. You had your doubts about some of them but in the end you knew they had to do the work, so you can't, it's not their fault, it's just they were there.

Source: www.open.ac.uk/hsc/ldsite/mabel/

This approach was influential. In the 1980s, for example, Graham Scambler explored how stigma could impact on people diagnosed with epilepsy. He suggested that being diagnosed with epilepsy as children results in a 'mindset' caused by over-protective adults which leads those with epilepsy to choose to conceal their diagnosis. However, it is this strategy which disrupts the lives of those with epilepsy, even more than any actual discrimination that occurs. For people who have been misdiagnosed, this can mean that the epilepsy 'label' might have more serious implications than any physical symptoms. From this perspective, being diagnosed with epilepsy could be seen as something of a personal tragedy (Scambler, 2004, 2011).

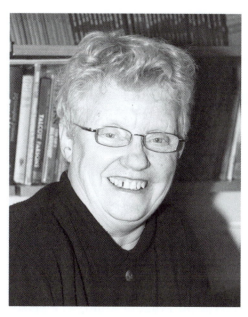

Figure 8.1 Mabel Cooper

Photograph courtesy of Dorothy Atkinson, Tanya Hames and Jane Abraham

Biographical Disruption and Personal Meaning

How individuals deal with stigma was of interest to Michael Bury who, like Scambler, was concerned with chronic illness, in particular, rheumatoid arthritis. Developing a chronic illness, Bury suggested, disrupts a person's knowledge about themselves and the world. It disrupts their understanding of day-to-day living. To maintain everyday life people therefore need to mobilize resources to repair the story of their lives (Bury, 1982). Bury's influential concept of **'biographical disruption'** has since been applied to cancer (Reeve et al., 2010), HIV, multiple sclerosis and chronic respiratory illness, to chronic illness with a sudden onset, such as hypoglycaemia among patients with diabetes mellitus, as well as stroke and motor neurone disease (Felde, 2011).

Biographical disruption: occurs when a person is forced to re-think who they are and where their life is going (their biography) as a result of being diagnosed with a chronic illness.

In Chapter 5, in the discussion about dying, it was suggested the experience of not being able to control our own bodies may shake our sense of personhood (Lawton, 2000). This view owes much to Kathy Charmaz, who herself suffered constant respiratory infections and haemorrhaging after a tonsillectomy as a child. Charmaz drew attention to issues of personal meaning. She challenged a narrow biomedical approach to chronic illness which defined illness solely in terms of physical discomfort. In particular, she argued that 'loss of self' is a powerful form of suffering for people who are chronically ill, leading them to live restricted lives, experience social isolation, be discredited and burden others (Charmaz, 1983).

By the 1990s, however, the kind of research about chronic illness pioneered by Scambler, Bury and Charmaz began to be criticized, in particular by those from the field of disability studies. Disability activists were concerned that a focus on stigma portrayed disabled people as 'the largely passive victims of stigma labels' (Barnes and Mercer, 2010: 51). They especially challenged the idea that disability is a personal tragedy. Whilst some disabled and chronically ill people may understand their experiences in these terms, many do not. The idea of disability as a personal tragedy can be viewed as a disabling social construct which may say more about the fears and prejudices of people who are not disabled, than about the realities of life as a disabled person. Sociologists today agree that many of the problems of chronically ill people are usefully understood through the same framework of oppression that informs the disability movement. As suggested in Chapter 7 on Sexuality, it is important to think about stigma as linked in to power inequalities in society, as something that is done *to* people. Graham Scambler himself has been important in emphasizing this view (Scambler, 2011: 36). A better focus is on wider society and how and why it causes inequality for disabled people.

In recent years, studies of chronic illness and disability have tended to draw together. The disability critique of biomedicine offers a way of looking at things which has also been valuable for people suffering from chronic illness, particularly when it comes to ensuring legal rights (Wendell, 2001). Carol Thomas, who interviewed cancer survivors, suggests that the damage done by cancer can mean that cancer survivors are vulnerable to **disablism**. Cancer continues to haunt their lives in the form of loss of employment, low income and financial problems into their later years and the reactions of others (Thomas, 2010: 50/1).

Disablism: discrimination or prejudice against people with disabilities.

The emphasis of much research in this area is on the 'cognitive' aspects of disability. Kathy Charmaz, for example, emphasizes the rational agency of people who are chronically ill as they remake their lives (1991, 2000). This emphasis has also drawn attention to the ways in which people resist stereotypes and stigma. Scambler, for example, has highlighted recently how a small minority of people with epilepsy 'resist or actively combat' stigmatizing constructions of their condition. Whilst almost all current (Western) stigma reduction programmes for epilepsy focus on the importance of education, the quality of life of those with epilepsy is a product of biological, psychological and social mechanisms. This makes the minority of people who have found a way to resist the epilepsy 'mind-set' very important

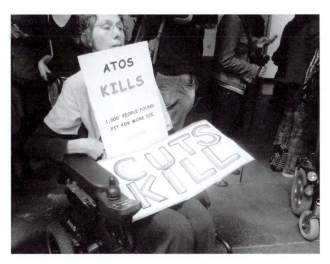

Figure 8.2 Disabled activist, London, 31 August, 2012, participating in a week of action called by DAC (Disabled People Against Cuts) and UK Uncut against Atos, a company selected by the Department of Work and Pensions to carry out controversial Work Capability Assessments, and sponsor of the Paralympic Games

Photograph courtesy of Corbis Images

(Scambler, 2011). Framed in this way, 'outsider' status can be a source of celebration and power, not just a source of suffering (see Figure 8.3). Just as LGBT activists have taken ownership of words like 'gay' and 'queer' and used them as a powerful source of identity and pride, disabled activists have also taken stigmatizing stereotypes and redrawn them. 'What the **** is normal?' asks comedian Francesca Martinez, who rejects the biomedical label 'cerebral palsy', preferring her own term, 'wobbly'.

Body Problems

One of the reasons why research has moved towards emphasizing the understanding and agency of chronically ill and disabled people themselves is because people researching disability are more likely today to be chronically ill or disabled. In recent years, the voices of people with learning disabilities have also begun to be heard in research about their conditions (Atkinson and Walmesley, 2010). But this involvement has also led to calls to 'reinstate' impairment in how disability is understood. Whilst an emphasis on discrimination is important, it is also clear that impairments themselves can be an enormous problem and source of grief and trauma (Hughes and Paterson, 1997). This shift also fits with a move towards understanding emotion, not just cognition. Attention has turned to how bodily experiences such as pain and emotions such as exhaustion may be as important in changing how people think of themselves as more cognitive processes (Reeve et al., 2010). For example, Frank (1995) suggested that experiencing chronic illness involves needing to tell a new story about the body, but the dominance of medical language means stories of the body are often 'unrecognized and invalidated'. This poses a problem for patients. If they adopt the biomedical language they can achieve recognition but at the expensive of becoming alienated from their own experience (see Case Study: Living with Chronic Pain). The increasingly common experience of multi-morbidity only highlights the challenges for individuals trying to make sense of and manage bodily problems (Pickard and Rogers, 2012).

....

CASE STUDY

Living with Chronic Pain

As many as one in five people in Europe suffers from chronic pain, only recognized as a disease since 2001. Maya Lavie-Ajayi and colleagues interviewed six men and women about their experiences of living with the condition. Their interviews show how the bodily problem of chronic pain also creates a unique emotional problem due to the failure of the medical discourse and wider society to acknowledge the condition. On the one hand, chronic pain is a vivid and total experience which affects every aspect of life: work, relationships and family. It can completely change a person's life and lead to frustration, disappointment and despair: 'I lost the will to live'. Yet the degree of pain also changes frequently and without warning. This elusive nature of chronic pain makes it difficult to convince family and friends and medical professionals, including those assessing their right to government benefits. These others may deny, conceal or delegitimize their experiences, suggesting that they are either pretending or exaggerating their condition, in turn provoking feelings of guilt, shame, anger and frustration:

> I came in and the doctor started touching my foot and I started crying and shouting, and he said 'come on, you are exaggerating!'... I am so furious with this, he really degraded me.

This pressure may lead sufferers to deny their own pain and lose trust in their own ability to judge their bodily sensations. Yet believing in the pain and proving that it exists also means accepting that they have a disability, an identity they may reject because they do not wish to be seen as 'abnormal'.

Source: Lavie-Ajayi, M. et al. (2012) 'Chronic pain as a narratological distress: a phenomenological study', *Chronic Illness*, 8(3): 192–200.

....

The burgeoning research on chronic illness and disability can be seen as reflecting an increase in the proportion of people in society whose have everyday problems relating to the functioning of their bodies. As Chapter 2 suggested, the rise of the 'worried well' demonstrates that the boundaries between those who are ill and those who are well are permeable. Frank (1995) suggests that we live in a 'remission society'. Those we think of as survivors include not only those who have experienced serious physical illness but also those recovering from substance abuse or mental illness. The stories of those who are managing ongoing physical conditions are a valuable resource for us all.

Implications for Practice

Health care practitioners enter into a relationship with a chronically ill or disabled person equipped with a body of expert knowledge, including biomedical knowledge. This expertise can be a vital resource for a chronically ill or disabled person. However, to be genuinely useful for someone who has a chronic illness or a disability, a professional needs to understand the social and psychological aspects of body problems, especially the implications of discrimination. It is especially important, therefore, to respect the way the individual service user understands their situation and what it is they want from the therapeutic relationship.

Summary

- People who have chronic illness and disability face numerous social barriers which endanger their wellbeing
- Stigma is an important issue for chronically ill and disabled people but is closely linked to social structures which reproduce disadvantage
- Chronically ill and disabled people are not passive victims but actively involved in making sense of their experiences and devising new ways to manage their condition

Exercise

Having read the chapter, make a list of as many examples of chronic illness and disability as you can think of. Going through your list, what do you see as the most important factors impacting on the lives of people with these conditions? What are the differences? What are the similarities?

Further Reading

Barnes, C. and Mercer, G. (2010) *Exploring Disability: A Sociological Introduction*. Second Edition. Cambridge: Polity.

Grant, G. et al. (eds) (2010) *Learning Disability: A Life Cycle Approach*. Second edition. Maidenhead, New York: McGraw-Hill/Open University Press.

Oliver, M. (2009) *Understanding Disability: From Theory to Practice*. Second Edition. London: Palgrave MacMillan.

Online readings

To access further resources related to this chapter, visit the companion website at www.sagepub.co.uk/russell

Fish, J. (2010) 'Promoting equality and valuing diversity for lesbian, gay, bisexual and trans patients', *InnovAiT*, 3(6): 333–38.

9

Mental health

Key issues

- Mental health involves social and psychological as well as biological factors
- The vulnerability of people to emotional distress reflects their experiences across the whole course of their lives
- Adversity is the major threat to mental health

Introduction

Chapter 1 discussed the biomedical approach to human health. It was suggested there that this approach, whilst offering a more scientific framework, tends to neglect the psychological and social aspects of human beings. Problems of the mind lie most obviously at the frontier between our biological lives and our cultural lives as members of society. The 'common sense' view of mental disorders today is that they are the result of a breakdown in the 'nerve centre' of our body 'machine' – the brain. That is, mental ill health is seen as a biological problem needing biomedical solutions such as drugs or surgery. However, a wealth of evidence suggests that whilst biology is of importance in matters of mental health, social environment is no less important. Difficult lives leave their marks on our human bodies but also on the state of our minds.

A Short History of Mental Illness

Evidence suggests that distress with no obvious external cause has been a challenge for all societies of which we have record. Those who believed in spirits and demons often saw mental disorder as a sign of possession and tried to use healing or ritual to release these negative influences (Millon, 2004). Trepanation, the drilling and removal of parts of the skull, for example, was practised throughout Neolithic times and is believed to have been carried out for 'magical, ritual and religious' reasons (Weber and Wahl, 2006: 537). From ancient sources onwards, two main approaches to treating mental illness can be identified: attempting to physically alter the body, especially the brain, and encouraging sufferers to talk (Sedgwick, 1982).

However, from the seventeenth century onwards, the idea that mental disorder could be explained by supernatural forces began to be challenged by the rise of a scientific approach to medicine which increasingly sought to find answers to mental distress by looking for bodily disorders (Foucault, 1965). Psychiatry, the wing of medicine dedicated to mental illness, eventually succeeded in dominating our understanding of emotional distress. However, the variety of different approaches in modern psychiatric practice is a sign that its biomedical focus did not go unchallenged. In the late nineteenth century, for example, Sigmund Freud, an Austrian neurologist, developed an extremely influential theory of human psychology, which rooted all emotional problems in childhood experience.

The biomedical search for the physiological origins of mental illness has not been a smooth one. In the early twentieth century psychiatry was very much associated with the eugenics movement (discussed in Chapters 4 and 8) which linked many kinds of social problems to genetic inferiority. Psychiatry was implicated in stigmatizing mental disorder by associating it with 'inbreeding' (De Bont, 2010: 151). During the First World War, biological explanations linking mental illness to underlying genetic vulnerability suddenly became highly problematic when, as a result of their experiences in warfare, a high proportion of troops, perhaps particularly those from the 'well-bred' officer class, experienced what is now known as 'Post Traumatic Stress Disorder'.

Nonetheless, the search for biomedical solutions to mental problems was far from discredited. Treatments developed in the 1930s such as insulin coma therapy, prefrontal lobotomy and electroconvulsive shock therapy could clearly bring some disorders to a dramatic halt, though these measures are now used much less widely, partly in recognition of the dramatic damage that they could also do. Twentieth-century neurological research expanded our understanding of mental disorder. It identified, for example, chemical imbalances of the brain associated with the mental disorder schizophrenia. Psychiatry regained influence and the introduction of major tranquillizers in the 1950s marked the beginning of an influential biomedical approach to treatment whose production, marketing and consumption has continued to expand, tending to reinforce the influence of psychiatry across the globe (Rogers and Pilgrim, 2010).

This short history highlights that mental disorder, like physical illness, is changing all the time (Healy, 2008). When circumstances 'break' people in the twenty-first century, the symptoms of our emotional suffering are expressed differently to the symptoms seen in other times. Diseases like 'hysteria' no longer exist (Scull, 2009), whilst depression has become a major disorder, suffered by more and more people around the world. Distress in the form of self-harm, anorexia nervosa, compulsive eating and other behaviours and many other disorders that exist today are quite recent historically.

Mental Health in Britain

One problem for those seeking to redress the suffering caused by mental illness is that the issue of defining mental health and illness is not straight-forward. Should mental health be measured by degree of happiness? By resilience in the face of hardship? Or should the focus be on unpleasant emotional symptoms, like hearing voices or feeling overwhelmed and unable to function? Even if the focus is on symptoms, assessing people in relation to others is not easy. Measuring mental distress presents special challenges as it involves subjective judgements about how we feel. One way to avoid these kinds of problems is to focus on behaviours rather than feelings and perceptions. What is the person doing that is causing trouble in their life or in the lives of others? Inevitably though, such a focus only leads us back to asking questions about our internal state.

Despite these problems, mental health is assessed in the same way we assess physical health, by identifying symptoms and comparing these with conditions identified by medical practitioners. These are listed in the *Diagnostic and Statistical Manual of Mental Disorders* produced by the American Psychiatric Association, whose fifth edition was published in May 2013 amidst great controversy, not least because of its expansion of signs and symptoms seen as signifying mental disorder (Scheid, 2013; Horwitz, 2002).

Disorders may then be grouped under headings such as 'common mental disorders' or 'anxiety disorders'. In Britain, for example, 17.6% of adults suffered from a common mental disorder in 2007 (ONS, 2011b: 27). The main disorder in this category is depression. In 2009/10 11.5% of people in Northern Ireland, 10.9% in England, 8.6% in Scotland and 7.9% in Wales experienced depression. Other disorders include generalized anxiety disorder, panic disorder, phobias and obsessive and compulsive disorders (OCD). Table 9.1, which presents data from England in 2004 and 2007, provides a sense of how common these disorders are.

Mental ill health represents 23% of the total British health bill yet accounts for nearly half of all ill health. Whilst one in four people in Britain will experience some kind of mental health problem in the course of a year, only one quarter of people who have a mental disorder are in treatment (LSE, 2012). Many who suffer anxiety and depression do not seek treatment and these diseases often go undiagnosed (NICE, 2011). It is also people of working age who are most affected by mental illness, which is responsible for nearly half of all absenteeism from work. Mental ill health also overlaps with physical ill health. One third of people with a physical illness will also have a mental illness and, in addition, a person who is depressed is 50% more disabled than a person suffering from angina, asthma, arthritis or diabetes (Moussavi et al., 2007).

Table 9.1 Percentage suffering from mental illness (England)

	% in population who are suffering	% of sufferers who are in treatment
Adults		
Schizophrenia or bipolar disorder	1	80
Depression and/or anxiety disorders		
Mainly depression	8	25
Mainly anxiety disorders	8	25
Any mental disorder	17	
Children (5–16)		
Conduct disorder or ADHD	6	28
Depression and/or anxiety disorders	4	24
Autistic Spectrum Disorder	1	43
Any mental disorder	10	

Source: LSE Centre for Economic Performance's Mental Health Policy Group (2012) *How Mental Illness Loses Out in the NHS*. London: London School of Economics: 7

Factors in Mental Illness

How are we to understand these serious conditions? Why do they happen and what is the best way to treat them? 'Common sense' understandings see mental illness as resulting from a malfunction of the brain, a 'bad' childhood or, in some cases, as no illness at all: 'some people are just evil'. As the following sections will show, moving beyond these understandings remains a challenge for us when trying to understand mental distress. Some of the major factors which will be considered here include: **social construction,** biology, **social class, urbanicity,** migration and **ethnicity, gender,** adversity across the life course and stigma and discrimination.

Is Mental Illness Socially Constructed?

The first factor to consider in relation to why mental illness occurs is social construction. The idea of social construction has been discussed throughout this book. I have suggested that many aspects of health which we tend to think of as biological in fact reflect social factors. The differences between 'races', for example, and between the personalities of men and women, as well as the state of our health at different ages, are not fixed in stone by genetic difference but reflect the influence of society. The same is true of mental health and illness. 'Madness' is not the same experience in every society. Anthropologists have mapped a variety of conditions experienced in various communities, which are not known in the developed world (Rosman et al., 2009: 74–75) (see Case Study: Idioms of Distress).

CASE STUDY

Idioms of Distress – Symptoms of Suffering Among the Quechua of Peru

Psychological distress is often associated with physical symptoms. However, the way we express and understand those physical symptoms, and even the way we experience them, reflects the culture we live in. Duncan Pedersen and his colleagues interviewed members of the Quechua community in the mountains of Peru. These villagers suffer extreme poverty and violence at the hands of the military. Many have witnessed the dismemberment of their loved ones. They told the researchers about the affects of these experiences. The villagers suffered from *pinsamientuwan* (worrying thoughts) and were afraid they would be killed as well. This problem could become so bad it resulted in *manan* (emptiness) or, its opposite, *tutal* (excess of thoughts). Both of these were considered serious and untreatable, equivalent to being *lukuyasca* (crazy, out of your mind). People who were *lukuyasca* could be identified by aimless walking, babbling speech, throwing stones against others, spilling food out of the pot, being dishevelled and going hatless to market (in a society where women in particular are always expected to wear a hat to market). The Quechua also use the term *llaki*, which refers to sadness and is associated with *ñakary* (suffering) – a life of worries caused by external causes such as material deprivation and insecurity. Extreme *llaki* can also result in *lukuyasca*. Both *llakil* and *ñakary* are associated with *umananay* (headache), *istumaguyki pawaspan* (stomach pain) and *wirpuypi malukuna* (body pains).

Source: Pedersen, D., Kienzler, H. and Gamarra, J. (2010) '*Llaki* and *Ñakary*: Idioms of distress and suffering among the Highland Quechua in the Peruvian Andes', *Culture, Medicine and Psychiatry*, 34: 279–300.

In 1960, Thomas Szasz, a Hungarian-born psychiatrist in New York, published an influential book called *Is Mental Illness a Myth?* Szasz argued that psychiatry was making a mistake in classifying mental distress in a biomedical frame, as 'illness'. He argued that by classifying those in distress as 'ill', psychiatrists were engaging in a **labelling** exercise which led to major changes in the lives of those so diagnosed. Having been told that they are 'mad', a person is increasingly treated in a particular way, which changes how they think about themselves and how they behave. By creating the label of 'mental illness', Szasz argued, psychiatry was operating as a powerful institution of social control (see Chapter 2), working to enforce social values about what is normal and appropriate behaviour (see Figure 9.1).

> Labelling: a process whereby a person who receives a diagnosis changes because of the changed reactions of other people to them.

These arguments and the 'anti-psychiatry' movement of which Szasz was a part, were important in challenging the idea that psychiatry is a neutral and objective science. Feminist authors have also highlighted ways in which a male-dominated psychiatric framework acted, in the nineteenth and twentieth century in particular, to pathologize women and their

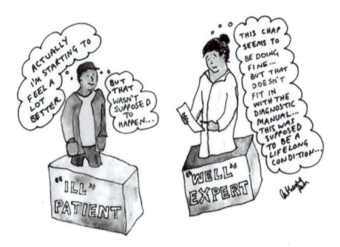

Figure 9.1   'Ill' Patient, 'Well' Expert: Cartoon by Catherine Pain

Copyright Open University. First appeared in Society Matters: http://www.open.ac.
uk/platform/blogs/society-matters

emotional disabilities, portraying the female psyche as inherently vulnerable and unstable (Bentley, 2005). Recent evidence even suggests that self-interested medical industries might be accused of consciously 'exporting' Western illness labels to the majority world, encouraging people to understand their distress in frameworks that are making them increasingly dependent on Western expertise and pharmacology (Watters, 2010).

However, there are several reasons to believe that mental illness is not simply created when a medical practitioner announces to a patient that they fall under a particular diagnostic label, as Szasz suggested in 1960. First, some symptoms of mental illness are physical, including lethargy and muscle pain, but also gastric ulcers and cardiovascular disease. Plainly, both the mind and the body are implicated in these diseases. Physical and emotional symptoms may exist and cause suffering long before a person presents themselves to a medical person for diagnosis. In addition, whilst we can recognize the potential for medical practitioners to pass off their personal prejudices as 'objective' judgements, when family members, workmates and friends notice that someone is not themselves, there is clearly something 'real' going on. For many people whose thoughts and emotions have been troubling them, receiving a diagnosis, care and treatment can be an enormous relief, rather than the beginning of a descent into irrationality (Rogers and Pilgrim, 2010: 3).

Moreover, despite the diversity of mental illness across the globe today and the need for more research to understand its different characteristics in different places, there are good reasons also to seek biological commonalities amongst people suffering from particular patterns of mental distress. Whilst conditions like schizophrenia appear to show more variety across the world than was previously thought (Morgan et al., 2008: 3) there do appear to be common symptoms underlying many conditions, notably depression (Rosman et al., 2009: 75).

Biology

What biological factors underlie mental distress? A great deal of attention has been directed to identifying problems such as chemical imbalances in the brain, and then to exploring the use of drugs or surgery to rectify those problems. In the past decade, genetic patterns have been of particular interest for those seeking a biological explanation. Interestingly, however, this research has revealed the importance of social factors creating the context in which a person's biological vulnerabilities may lead to emotional problems.

For example, until recently, the dominant view of schizophrenia was that it is a genetic brain disease. Social factors might trigger that disease, but its main cause was seen as biological. However, this view is changing (Morgan et al., 2008: 4). Researchers have found that a person's risk of developing psychosis as an adult is significantly influenced by events in their childhood, in particular, whether they have been exposed to adversity as children. Adverse events include losing a parent, or being separated from them for a long time, being in institutional care, being abused sexually, physically or emotionally, being neglected, bullied, or experiencing domestic violence or parental mental illness (Alemany et al., 2012; Varese et al., 2012).

Research suggests that these experiences have an impact on the body in the form of the functioning of the hypothalamus, pituitary, and adrenal glands, which work together (the 'HPA axis') to regulate many body processes. If a person experiences persistent stress in childhood this may raise levels of certain hormones in this biological feedback system which damages the system, making it overly sensitive to future stress. This over-sensitivity may also be related to problems involving the brain chemical dopamine, which is implicated in schizophrenia (Myin-Germeys and van Os, 2008).

This research is leading to a greater interest in social and psychological factors which influence mental health (some of these will be discussed in the following sections). Nonetheless, a biomedical approach remains dominant, for a number of reasons. One reason is that the prestige of psychiatry as a wing of medicine has depended on its ability to establish a clear biomedical justification for its existence. If mental problems are seen as primarily a social, not a medical problem, then the authority of psychiatry is reduced.

Another influential factor is the global pharmaceutical industry. Evidence suggests that drugs may be of limited help to many people suffering mental illness, and the benefits may be modest at best compared with placebos. Some drugs which continue to be widely prescribed and consumed have serious negative effects. Nonetheless, the pharmaceutical industry is expanding its influence (Kirsch, 2010). In England, for example, use of antidepressant medications rose 334% between 1991 and 2009, and in the course of the first eight or nine years of this century rates rose 88% in Wales, 54% in Scotland and 60% in Northern Ireland (ONS, 2011b: 29). Pharmaceutical companies develop new and supposedly 'better' drugs in response to research revealing the dangers of earlier brands, whilst also funding research aimed at identifying new frontiers for the **medicalization** of mental illness (Scull, 2009; Healy, 2008).

Two other influences are also worthy of mention. The use of drugs in mental illness can be dated back to the 1950s. The rise of this form of treatment broadly coincided with (but did not cause) (Rogers and Pilgrim, 2010) a shift towards caring for mentally ill people in the community rather than in institutions. Statistically, mentally ill people in the community are rarely dangerous. However, a variety of social forces have fuelled anxiety about tragic episodes where mentally ill people have taken the lives of strangers (see Case Study: Mental Health, Dangerousness and the Media). Tranquillizers, however unhelpful they may be for making people well, are one way of ensuring that these events can never happen, which may be another reason for their continued popularity. Finally, a drug is a consumer item which can be purchased by an individual seeking to take control of their mental health, an approach which has a particular appeal in a society which promotes both individualistic solutions and consumerism (Teghtsoonian, 2009). These arguments highlight that biological problems always occur in a social context. Social factors are important in understanding why one person experiences ongoing mental distress, whilst another does not. Important social factors include class, urbanicity and migration, adversity across the **life course**, gender, age, stigma and discrimination.

CASE STUDY

Mental Health, Dangerousness and the Media

The idea that mentally ill people are potentially dangerous and a risk to themselves and others is a popular theme increasingly reinforced in the media. However, the dangerousness of mental disorder should not be exaggerated. For example, most diagnoses such as 'schizophrenia' tell us little about a person's propensity for violence. A much better predictor of violence is substance abuse. Nonetheless, a clear pattern has emerged since the 1990s where emotional media coverage of rare and frightening incidents of violence has fuelled public anxiety about the risk of having mentally ill people in the community. The result has been pressure to change health policy to ensure that the focus of mental health workers is on assessing and managing the risks that mentally ill people pose to the public. Whilst random violence committed by mentally ill people does occur, this focus has had negative consequences for the civil liberties of mentally ill people, their wellbeing and how they think about themselves. For professionals working in health and social care it makes their jobs more stressful and means being required to 'police' service users rather than care for them. For society at large, arguably, this over-emphasis on dangerousness feeds stigma about mental illness and increases our everyday levels of anxiety and perceptions of danger which might even contribute to higher levels of mental illness.

Sources: Hewitt, J.L. (2008) 'Dangerousness and mental health policy', *Journal of Psychiatric and Mental Health Nursing*, 15: 186–94; Cummins, I. (2010) 'Distant voices, still lives: reflections on the impact of media reporting of the cases of Christopher Clunis and Ben Silcock', *Ethnicity and Inequalities in Health and Social Care*, 3(4): 18–29.

Social Factors in Mental Illness: Class, Urbanicity and Migration

In 1939, two US researchers noticed that rates of mental illness, especially schizophrenia, depended on where people in Chicago were living. The highest rates were in places that were socially disorganized, characterized by poverty, crime and poor housing. Today, it is well established that social disadvantages produce mental health disadvantages (McLeod, 2013). The class gradient (see Chapter 3) is most striking in relation to schizophrenia and least clear in relation to affective disorders, but exists for most diagnoses. Evidence also suggests that mental health professionals judge and treat people differently according to their class (Smith, 2005).

In addition to social class, two other major factors implicated in mental ill health are urbanicity and migration. A strong and consistent finding is that the risk for schizophrenia increases with the number of years spent living in a city (McKenzie, 2008) and there is evidence that this effect may even stronger for those born more recently (Krabbendam, 2005). Mood and anxiety orders such as depression are also higher in urban areas (Peen et al., 2010). The precise reason why cities are dangerous in this way is not clear. It may be due to the faster pace and stressfulness of everyday life, the concentration of poverty in urban areas or greater differentiation of people resulting in poor social integration. One characteristic of people with mental illness is that their social networks are more restricted. Their networks may be only 20–30% as extensive as others, with a third having no friends at all (Warner, 2008: 173). It is unlikely that the problem with cities can be explained in relation to just one factor. A combination of factors is probably involved including housing, work, family problems and security (Wang, 2004). Some evidence also suggests that living in a rural area can also lead to mental health problems, and it is possible that mental health suffers in both extreme rural and urban areas (Walters et al., 2004).

> Urbanicity: the impact of living in an urban area at a given time, taking into account that there may be degrees to which an environment can be described as urban depending on factors such as population density.

A striking finding is that migration increases a person's risk of developing schizophrenia (Craig, 2011: 107). Evidence suggests that this is particularly true for dark-skinned migrants living in countries where the majority have white skin. For example, in Britain, low levels of educational attainment and employment, poor housing, living alone and being without long-term relationships, as well as deprivation and social isolation, are consistently more common amongst black African Caribbean patients (see also Case Study 'African Caribbean Psychosis in Britain' in Chapter 4) (Cantor-Graae and Selten, 2005). The relationship between migration and depression is less clear. Rates may be different for different migrant groups and vary according to their migrant status. Whilst it is clear that migration is 'very stress-inducing', different migrants have different experiences, and coping strategies and resilience are factors in migrant mental health (Bhugra, 2004). Some research also suggests that in some contexts ethnicity may protect mental health (Mossakowski, 2003).

Adversity Across the Life Course

All of the social factors discussed so far can usefully be thought about in relation to a life perspective approach to mental health which considers the impact of adversity across the life course. The idea of accumulation of risk of physical illness over the course of our lives, introduced in the chapter on ageing, is also very relevant to mental illness. The idea that early childhood experiences might affect our mental health dates back to the founder of psychoanalysis, Sigmund Freud. In the 1960s, radical youth movements created a context in which it became fashionable to blame 'bad parenting' for social problems (Hinshaw, 2005). Later generations of researchers recoiled from these approaches which failed to consider the impact on parents of the wider social circumstances in which they are attempting to parent. More recent research takes a less judgemental approach to understanding the impact on children of adversity and trauma in childhood, including parental neglect and hostility, sexual and physical abuse. It is clear that early adversity does increase the risk of psychosis in later life. In addition, this risk accumulates over time. Those exposed to harm when they are young are at greater risk of psychosis when they are older, and their vulnerability increases if they also experience risk factors such as migration, urbanicity or cannabis use (Alemany et al., 2012; Varese et al., 2012).

Researchers have made some effort to identify exactly what kind of adversity is most dangerous. Holmes and Rahe (1967) for example, developed an inventory of significant life events that might be damaging. In 1978, Brown and Harris conducted an influential study of depressed women in London using an interview method. They identified life events and difficulties which might have an impact on a person's life including changes in their role such as losing a job or finding a new partner, major changes in household roles, major health changes, moving house, receiving bad news or witnessing a serious accident (Brown, 1989). Their research strongly suggested that the meaning of negative life events is not fixed but must be understood in the context of an individual's life as a whole. Subsequent research also suggests that small, daily stresses of life may be more significant than rarer, major events like losing a parent or a job (Grzywacz et al., 2004).

Gender and Age

A person's early life experiences will then combine with later experiences and other social factors to influence their vulnerability to anxiety or psychosis. For example, there is evidence that women are more vulnerable to mental illness than men, but age is also important. In 2007 13.6% of men and 21.5% of women had experienced a 'common mental disorder' in the previous week. For example, women suffered more from anxiety and depression (ONS, 2011b). One reason for this finding may be that doctors are more prone to diagnose depression in women, even when using standardized measures. Stereotypes appear to operate, for example, predisposing doctors to diagnose emotional problems in women and alcohol problems in men (Afifi, 2007: 386). Yet there are good reasons why women might be vulnerable to depression. As suggested in Chapter 6, women are more likely to be victims of violence than men. On the other hand, psychoses, mental disorders that involve delusions, hallucinations and other problems of thought and emotion, are fairly rare but perhaps more common amongst men (McGrath et al., 2004; McManus et al., 2009). Males over 15 in the UK are also three times more likely than women to commit suicide (ONS, 2013c).

However, gender differences cannot be understood independently of age differences. Researchers found recently that in England after the age of 45 there is no significant difference in rates of psychosis between men and women. Moreover, for affective psychoses (which include bipolar disorder) rates were similar until age 45, after which women had significantly higher rates. It is suggested that prior to this time, oestrogen has a broadly protective effect for women, which is lost after menopause. However, changes in women's lives and expectations at this time are also implicated (Kirkbride et al., 2011: 156). Age is also important in relation to suicide rates, as it is men in the age group 30 to 44 who are particularly at risk in Britain (ONS, 2013c).

Stigma and Discrimination

It is clear that both biological and social factors are involved in mental illness. One particular social factor, however, deserves further mention. Whilst we may not agree with Szasz that mental illness is simply a myth, a state imposed on patients by psychiatry, the label of being 'mentally ill' clearly does involve stigma and discrimination which changes the lives of people who receive this diagnosis in negative ways. Thomas Scheff (1966) developed 'labelling theory' to explain the dynamics of mental illness. He suggested that a person diagnosed by a psychiatrist as mentally ill is then subject to stereotyping and differential treatment, as a result of which, Scheff suggested, the label of being 'mad' might lead the person to break even more social rules. As explored in Chapters 7 and 8, Erving Goffman, in an extremely influential book, described this negative labelling as 'stigma' (Goffman, 1963).

A great deal of research has explored the impact of stigma on people with mental illness. Levels of knowledge about mental illness remain very low. Some evidence suggests attitudes have improved recently, together with what people say about how they would treat someone with a mental illness. However, unfortunately the evidence does not suggest these good intentions are reflected in better behaviour (Evans-Lacko et al., 2013). Clearly, stigma and discrimination are closely related. Stigma follows discrimination which disadvantages the mentally ill and increases the difficulties in their lives in some fundamental ways, for example, by making it more difficult for those with mental illness to find work, decent accommodation and supporting social networks. Discrimination can be devastating for relationships, including with children, for education, employment and housing with the consequence that, as with other disabilities, discrimination can mean greater disadvantage for the mentally ill than the condition itself (Thornicroft, 2006).

Unfortunately, discrimination also results in inferior healthcare. For example, family doctors and professionals trained to deal with mentally ill service users may be a principle source of stigma and pessimism about the possibility of recovery (Thornicroft et al., 2007; Ross and Goldner, 2009). It has been suggested that psychosis can be linked to 'social defeat', which may involve multiple discriminations, where individuals disadvantaged by migration status, ethnicity, poverty, disability or other factors find themselves 'defeated' every day in their interactions with other people (Whitley, 2011). Mental illness, from this perspective, should be considered a disability and efforts made to promote the provision of safe environments that protect mental health.

Implications for Practice

It is clear that good mental health is closely related to good physical health. However, as with physical disease, some of the most important factors affecting mental illness are social. Stigma and discrimination are clearly important issues for health and social care practitioners, who may themselves struggle with anxieties about working with people who are mentally ill because of socially constructed stereotypes portraying them as dangerous or anti-social. Promoting good mental health requires us to work sympathetically with individuals to help them to optimize their condition. It means being aware of the ways in which a variety of social circumstances may combine to put stress on any of us, but especially on those made vulnerable by previous hardship and adversity.

Summary

- Mental illness as we know it is a product of society
- A variety of social factors combine to jeopardize the mental health of individuals
- Health care professionals have a particular responsibility not to perpetuate stigma and discrimination against mentally ill service users

Exercise

1. Over the course of a week, observe and make a note of any media portrayals of mentally ill people you can find. These may be in newspaper articles, radio or television announcements or programmes, films, YouTube clips or commentary on blogs, Facebook or Twitter, including jokes.
2. Consider your notes. How does the evidence you have found demonstrate points made in this chapter?

Further Reading

Busfield, J. (2011) *Mental Illness. Key Concepts.* Cambridge: Polity Press.

Rogers, A. and Pilgrim, D. (2010) *A Sociology of Mental Health and Illness.* Fourth edition. Maidenhead: Open University Press.

WHO publications on mental health at: www.who.int/mental_health/evidence/en/

 Online readings

To access further resources related to this chapter, visit the companion website at www.sagepub.co.uk/russell

Scheid, T.L. (2013) 'A decade of critique: notable books in the sociology of mental health and illness', *Contemporary Sociology: A Journal of Reviews* 42(2): 177–83.

10

Health care

Key issues

- Health care work occurs in a social context
- Key themes include **neoliberalism**, **bureaucracy**, **managerialism**, account-ability, community care and participation
- These themes reflect the **globalization** of health care

Introduction

A number of chapters in this book have offered insight about the health of particular sub-groups of health care service users: ethnic minority people, older people and those with mental health needs, for example. You may have wondered as you have read these chapters whether sociology can shed any light on the challenges of working in this sector. What does sociology mean for you in your future profession, whether you are training as a doctor, nurse or podiatrist, an occupational therapist or a radiographer? As well as studying health patterns, sociologists have been interested to study health care professionals and the wider environments in which they work. This chapter introduces some of the organizations, policies and contexts that have been associated with the paid provision of care in our society.

A Short History of Paid Care

As described in Chapter 1, prior to the nineteenth century, health care, as we now know it in Britain, did not exist. If health problems developed, people were cared for by those closest to them, or they visited some kind of village healer. Whilst there were physicians – members of the clergy who were experts in the 'healing arts' – that profession was very different to the one we know today. For example, in the thirteenth century physicians were forbidden by the Catholic Church from performing surgery, as it was believed that contact with blood or body fluids would contaminate their souls. Cutting the body was considered a craft, and carried out by a class of barbers. Over time, 'barber surgeons' developed their skills and organized themselves in competition with physicians (see Figure 10.1). In the sixteenth century they established an agency to regulate training and certification of surgical practice (Bagwell, 2005). Though surgery as we know it did not develop until antiseptics and anaesthetics were developed in the nineteenth century this was a step towards a scientific approach to all medicine, not just surgery. The image shows a barber surgeon tending a peasant's foot. We see few of the items associated with surgery today: white coats, gloves and carefully disinfected instruments. Rather, the barber surgeon wears everyday clothing, as does his customer, and the procedure is carried out on the floor of his workshop, illustrating unawareness of the danger of germs. Behind him, on the wall, are displayed an assortment of tools suggestive of the broad range of tasks a barber surgeon might be called upon to perform: a saw, what appears to be a crossbow, a brace.

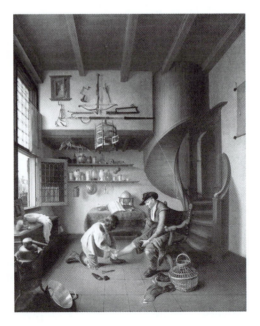

Figure 10.1   Isaack Koedijck. *Barber surgeon tending a peasant's foot* (c. 1649–50), oil on panel

This is the story of just one group of health care professionals, whose occupation went from being semi-skilled to the high paid, high status job that surgery is today. This example is valuable because it demonstrates how the status and fortunes of a professional group can change enormously over time, due largely to the efforts of those in the profession. This example also serves as an early model of the process by which other professions came into being.

For modern doctors, the turning point was in 1858. The Medical Act of that year established a basis for telling the difference between a qualified and an unqualified doctor and required doctors to be registered in order to practice. This Act established that doctors themselves were to be the judge of what was meant by medical expertise. With the rise of hospitals, doctors needed people to assist them. By the early twentieth century, the women who played this role had succeeded in establishing their own profession and rules for entrance with the 1919 Nurses Registration Act. Other professional groups followed a similar pattern.

The profession of physiotherapy, for example, came about when those offering massage for therapeutic purposes realized they needed to distance themselves from prostitution. Scandals about massage work in the 1890s led to the formation of the Society of Trained Masseuses who developed a model of practice to set rules about contact between the therapist and the patient. As part of this project, they adopted a biomechanical model of physical rehabilitation. By associating themselves with the idea that the body is a machine rather than a sensual being, they laid the basis for physiotherapy to become a legitimate wing of **biomedicine** (Nicholls and Cheek, 2006).

Other health professions that exist today have their own histories. Their rise reflected the growing credibility of biomedicine but also wider changes in society associated with industrialization, especially a new concern amongst emerging elites about the management and regulation of national populations (Foucault, 1975). The twentieth century saw a proliferation of professional groups in the area of health and social care, a product of the increasing complexity of efforts to ensure the health of the labour force.

Health Care Professionals

'Common sense' tells us that a health care professional is a person employed in a skilled and trustworthy occupation. The idea of 'professionalism' is associated with someone who knows what they are doing and has high ethical standards. However, as the short history above shows, the professions are, as much as biomedicine, gender or age, a product of society. They have a history and evolve in a wider social context. To understand why professionals behave the way they do and the pressures on them, we need to consider where the professions came from and the direction they are going.

One way to understand the professions is to see them as an essentially positive product of a modernizing, more rational society. The sociologist Émile Durkheim viewed professions as cohesive communities based on shared ethical values, giving them a special moral role as industrializing societies became more specialized (Gabe et al., 2004: 164). From this perspective, health professionals exist because they have a function in society. This is certainly a view that accords with the way professionals like to see themselves: that every characteristic of their group exists because this is what society needs from them. There are, however, clear problems with this 'common sense' view of professions. For example, tensions are common between members of different professions because of competing interpretations of the purpose and value of their work. Those who are not professionals may be even more critical. So to understand professionalism in a meaningful way requires a more distanced, sociological approach.

The sociologist Eliot Friedson (1975), though a supporter of the professions, suggested that one of their main characteristics is that they are a group of employees who achieve legitimate, organized autonomy. That is, other people need to be convinced that these individuals should be allowed to take responsibility for this area of knowledge and practice. To achieve this legitimacy in the eyes of others, they need long training in a body of specialist knowledge and a service orientation. Professions like nursing and midwifery and others achieved the status of professions by following the course taken by the medical profession.

This view suggests professional status is something that has to be worked for by a group of employees and achieved over time. Other writers in the 1970s were more critical. The Marxist Terry Johnson, for example, suggested that professions like medicine represent an institutionalized form of social control (1972). He argued that the power of professionals stems from the gap between the service user's lack of knowledge and the specialist knowledge of the professional expert. Feminist thinkers also developed the idea of professions as institutions of social control whilst highlighting the issue of gender. They suggested that professions were one way men maintained their dominance in society. For example, the rise of the medical profession, mostly male in the first part of the twentieth century, was associated with the marginalization of mostly female midwives. The **medicalization** of childbirth (see Chapter 2, Power) was therefore a process controlled by men (Oakley, 1980). Similarly, the low pay and status of nursing reflected the low status of women in society as well as the low status of work associated with 'women's role', work such as looking after other people, preparing food and cleaning. The nurses, midwives and radiographers in Britain who struggled to achieve and defend their professional status were therefore also challenging the low status of women (Witz, 1992).

Others have suggested, however, that the very idea of a professional is a product of women's inequality. For one group to reserve the most complicated work for themselves they need to have other people who will be left to do the mundane, less attractive jobs. Women themselves have recognized this and tried to escape from dirty or boring work. Nurses, for example, increased their status by making university training a requirement, emulating doctors. This achievement created the need for a new and growing group of workers called Health Care Assistants, who do the jobs that nurses will no longer do (see Case Study: 'We are the ones that wipe the bum'). By this argument, a real challenge to gender inequality needs to address the low status of certain types of work, rather than simply seek to move some women out of those jobs (Davies, 1995).

··

'We are the ones that wipe the bum' – Health Care Assistants and Nurses

The nursing profession was successful in making university education a requirement for registration. One outcome of this has been the growing number of Health Care Assistants (HCAs). HCAs work under the supervision of nurses, performing tasks nurses may no longer perform, such as washing patients. These different roles are reflected in 'boundary work' by both nurses and HCAs. Researchers spoke to employees at two acute NHS trusts in England about the differences. Nurses they spoke to emphasized the value of their qualifications in comparison to HCAs: 'You've got somebody there who's had 3 years of training... they've got accountability, they're trained...' HCAs, on the other hand, prided themselves on spending more time with patients: 'they trust you and they will tell you anything', whilst also being aware of being expected to do the 'dirty' work: 'We are the ones that wipe the bum, when it's very, very difficult and smelly... they call the HCAs, you know'. HCAs interviewed resented being prevented from doing some tasks because they are not qualified. They also resented the reaction they provoked if they 'overstepped' their role, for example, by pointing out poor nursing practice. For nurses, under pressure to complete paper work and other tasks, it could seem that HCAs did not understand the complexity of their work and its value for patients. Yet closeness to

(Continued)

(Continued)

patients is at the core of nursing identity, a feature of nursing that nurses have seen as marking them out from doctors. Many nurses expressed anxiety at becoming distanced from direct patient care.

Source: Bach, S. et al. (2009) 'Nursing a grievance? The role of healthcare assistants in a modernized National Health Service', *Gender, Work and Organization* 19(2): 205–23.

··

This important feminist work offered a new perspective on the challenges facing professional groups trying to improve their status in society. From the 1980s, however, sociologists found that what needed to be explained was not the power of medical professionals but the ways in which they were losing power. In various ways, medical professions have been forced to respond to an environment in which their status and authority has increasingly been brought into question (Gabe et al., 2004: 167). The following sections will consider some important themes of the social policy environment in which professional health care work is carried out in Britain today. These include neoliberalism, bureaucracy, managerialism, accountability, community care and participation.

Social Policy: Neoliberalism

Social policy refers to the actions, laws and principles that affect the living conditions of people in society. Social policy both influences and is influenced by trends in health and health care. There is a 'back and forth' relationship between laws and policies and what is happening in society, with each influencing the other. Social policy also both reflects and influences the power of particular groups in society (see Chapter 2). In particular, an essential feature of the context for social policy has been the state of the economy. In recent decades social policy, in all areas of government responsibility, has been profoundly influenced by the doctrine of neoliberalism.

Prior to the establishment of National Insurance in 1911 and the National Health Service in 1948, people who could not find employment or lived on low incomes were in a very vulnerable position, especially if they became unwell. The philosophy behind those reforms was to try to redress this inequality and to protect those negatively affected by economic forces outside of their control, such as recession. The introduction of the NHS brought immediate improvements to the health of the population in the years following the Second World War. This was a time when people were enthusiastic about the benefits to society of rational planned state control of the economy. However, it was also a time when economies worldwide were buoyant, a situation which did not last.

By the late 1970s concerns about the problem of finding funding for public health were gathering strength in the context of problems in the global economy. The Thatcher Conservative Government elected in 1979 was motivated by a 'neoliberal' philosophy. They believed the best way to provide resources in society was to minimize the role of **the state** in the economy whilst giving private companies freedom to invest in any production that would create profit. The argument was that if something was valuable to society, there would be demand for it and if there was demand for it, people would be willing to pay for it. If they could not pay for it, they would be motivated by the absence of state support to find ways to improve their situation. Even after that Government lost power to the Blair Labour Government in 1997, neoliberalism continued to be a powerful influence on government policy.

Neoliberalism: a political approach which favours minimal government intervention in business and reducing spending on welfare.

Neoliberal policies have shaped the environment in which health professionals work for over 30 years. Whilst in previous years doctors in particular were able to resist changes they did not like, from the 1990s the medical professions have struggled to maintain their conditions and the quality of their work under the impact of reforms designed to make health care dependent on economic markets. For example, in 1990 hospitals and other health care providers were made into Trusts, public corporations independent of health authorities. The idea was to make health and social services market products. Trusts would be motivated to provide health care that was good quality but also cost efficient. There would be less public money spent on health and families and individuals would respond to this by taking more responsibility for their own health.

The Labour Government elected in 1997 were also committed to encouraging private companies to invest in health to reduce the burden on taxation. Though they at first reduced the freedom of the Trusts, their power soon began to be re-established. The Blair Government also offered companies the opportunity to build private hospitals, in partnership with the state, accruing large long-term debts in the process. From the 1990s health care also saw control of resources devolved, greater community-based provision and an emphasis on the patient as 'consumer'.

However, there was much criticism of this approach. It has been argued that saving money is being given a higher priority than patient care, increasing waiting lists and leading to errors. In 1999, Scotland, Wales and Northern Ireland were given control of many areas of government, including health, and this led to Scotland and, to a lesser extent, Wales, moving away from a market-driven approach. In England, shutting of care homes by councils and contracting of care work to private companies has been associated with a growing crisis of care for older people (Bennett, 2012).

Bureaucracy and Managerialism

Two further social policy themes relevant to care work today are bureaucracy and managerialism. A useful starting point is to consider what the German philosopher Max Weber (see Chapter 3, Class) wrote about bureaucracy. Indeed, it was Weber who brought this word, now widely used, into our thinking. Weber offered a corrective to Karl Marx, arguing that in addition to class, a person's status is also important and relevant to their position in society. Weber was particularly interested in the changing world of work in the early twentieth century. What he noticed was the way in which rationality, that defining feature of **the Enlightenment** and the rise of biomedicine, began to change everything. More and more, people responded to challenges by taking a rational, scientific approach, rather than a spontaneous, emotional approach as they had in the past.

One result of this was the development of more and more rules governing the right and wrong way to do things. Where previously people decided what to do in a fairly instinctive way, based on past practice, they now sought the advice of competent experts who provided impersonal procedures for non-experts to follow. The more rules there were, the more there also developed hierarchies to ensure that rules agreed by a small group of people would be followed by everyone. Those at the top were responsible for ensuring that those in the next rung of the hierarchy were following the rules, and so on down through a pyramid of responsibility. In this way, bureaucracy increasingly spread throughout workplaces and government bodies. For Weber, this meant that the hold of rational organization on our modern society was becoming like an 'iron cage' (Weber, 1978).

> Bureaucracy: the hierarchical administration of an organization by a body of non-elected officials.

Many other writers since Weber have explored the ways in which bureaucratic institutions have worked to keep control of people at the bottom of the hierarchy. Much evidence also shows, however, that modern bureaucracies are not the paragons of iron rationality implied by Weber's description. For example, the sociologist Peter Blau (1963) showed that informal channels are essential to the functioning of a bureaucracy. Employees bending rules that are too rigid actually helps organizations to function.

Nonetheless, our society is not moving away from rules and bureaucracy towards spontaneity. The public sector and health care institutions such as the NHS, for example, have become more and more bureaucratic. The growth of bureaucracy has been criticized because of its cost to taxpayers. Closely associated to this greater bureaucracy is a growing layer of managers, whose importance in the system is a product of managerialism.

Managerialism is the idea that any matter of organization can be managed according to rational procedures to achieve aims defined by senior management. For example, the role of managers is to run businesses more efficiently to save money and to motivate people to want to work hard. From at least the 1980s, managers have been influential in the public as well as the private sector, associated with neoliberal ideas that public bodies should be run more like businesses. For example, management consultants Osborne and Gaebler (1992, cited in Cooke and Philpin, 2008: 54–5) argued that market competition could reduce the amount of bureaucracy in the public sector. However, whilst the number of clinical staff in the NHS rose 32% between 1998 and 2008, the number of managers rose by 76% (Vize, 2009, cited in Jarman and Greer, 2010a).

Managerialism: the application of managerial techniques to running non-business organisations like the civil service and local authorities.

The rise of managers and of bureaucracy is also associated with concerns that professionals cannot be trusted to regulate poor performance within their own ranks (Traynor et al., 2013). It was argued that if managers were 'free to manage' they could regulate professionals who had failed to regulate themselves. A series of medical scandals created a focus on unethical professional behaviour. For example, in the 1990s it was found that doctors had been secretly keeping organs from dead children with-out the consent of parents, the first of a series of similar episodes. In 2000, GP Harold Shipman was found guilty of murdering 15 patients and a subsequent report found he had probably killed 250 people. Tighter regulation and more rules followed. However, it has been suggested that the introduction of more and more rigid rules about procedures is alien-ating for staff and patients (Ritzer, 1996; Sennett, 2008). The tendency for senior managers to seek continual change to procedures to respond to indicators of inefficiency does not help. In recent years this has led to a call for more 'leadership' to bridge the gap of mistrust between profes-sionals and managers (O'Reilly and Reed, 2010).

Accountability

The rise of bureaucracy and managerialism is associated with concern about accountability. When mistakes are made and the health of patients is compromised, will someone be held to account? As suggested in Chapter 1 (Biomedicine), where once the authority of biomedical experts, resting in their scientific qualifications, was unquestioned, this is no longer true. Lay people know more about health and how to manage their own health. They anticipate health risks, are better able to find out information for themselves and are more likely to challenge medical experts. Concerns about well-publicised episodes of poor standards of care, notably at Stafford Hospital in England, have led to calls for an end to self-regulation and a 'new profes-sionalism' (Gabe and Calnan, 2009; Light, 2003). Nurses, once portrayed in a very positive way in the media, have also increasingly been the subject of attention due to poor performance (Traynor et al., 2013) (see Case Study: 'I don't know what's wrong with these people').

'I don't know what's wrong with these people': failures of care

A sociological approach to patient safety emphasizes the importance of understanding the social context in which failures of care occur. Alexandra Hillman and colleagues spent time in acute hospital trusts in England, closely studying how risk is managed on the wards. Their research highlights the development of a culture of defensiveness about safety which leads staff to view patients as an enemy against whom they must defend themselves. Notes from a member of the research team illustrate this:

> Two members of staff [...] come up to the nurses' station and ask Jim (a Staff Nurse) about Fred, a man on the ward who'd had a fall. He tells them that Fred said he'd fallen 'but he was back in bed and given how much he struggles in and out of bed I don't know how he would've got himself back into bed'. [...] Jackie (an Health Care Assistant) tells me, 'Fred says he had a fall out of the bed onto the floor right but he never could've got off the floor if that'd happened'.
>
> Jim: He did say this morning that he almost fell.
>
> Jackie: That's why no-one will see to him on their own now.
>
> Jim: It's turned into a big game of them and us.

The authors argue that anxiety about safety has created a disconnection between staff and patients that threatens the provision of dignified care:

> Jackie goes to do some observations on the bay and Fred is really pulling at his incontinence pad, catheter and pyjama bottoms. She goes back and asks Amy to come and help her and they pull the curtains round. I then hear her shout 'No, you've got to keep them on' followed by 'No, no no!'
>
> She comes out from behind the curtain and throws it back behind her in anger. As she goes by me she says 'why do they insist on digging' (earlier Jackie and Amy talked about patients they called 'gardeners' referring to those who go 'digging' inside their incontinence pads).

(Continued)

(Continued)

> I hear her tell her colleagues that 'he's put his hands in his pad and it's all
> over his sheets'. She has more sheets and a pad in her hand and as she goes
> by me again she looks at me and says 'I don't know what's wrong with
> these people. They start out in this world like babies and end up like babies'.

Source: Hillman, A., Tadd, W., Calnan, S., Bayer, A. and Read, S. (2013) 'Risk, governance and the experience of care', *Sociology of Health and Illness*. Early View.

Efforts to integrate health and social care as well as public concern about
professional malpractice have resulted in a particular focus on interprofessional teams. This focus is not confined to Britain. Research has highlighted
that failures of care can often be explained by failures in team working. For
example, in the United States, communication failure among team members
is a contributory factor in 60% of situations where a patient is killed or
injured due to an unanticipated event in a healthcare setting (Martin et al.,
2010:1). Worldwide initiatives to educate health and social care practitioners
at university in interprofessional teams from the outset (interprofessional
education, or IPE) represent an attempt to radically reshape the boundaries
between professions (see Figure 10.2).

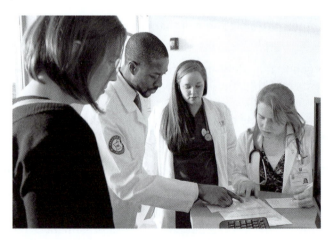

Figure 10.2   Interprofessional learning, Brown University, Providence, US
Photograph courtesy Mike Cohea/Brown University

Community Care

For centuries, many people with ongoing health issues or disabilities were placed in institutions where they lived out their whole lives. By the 1960s, those institutions were being closed on the basis that it would be better for those people to live in the community. The sociologist Erving Goffman (see Chapter 9, Mental Health) was influential in arguing that institutions are a form of social control and not in the best interests of service users. In addition, by the 1980s a series of scandals about the treatment of people living in long-stay mental health institutions, together with growing recognition of the rights of mentally ill people, led to more and more patients being discharged. Small group homes began to be provided under the slogan 'care in the community'. However, because of attempts to cut back on public spending, by the 1980s it was clear that care was being provided *by* the community, not just *in* it.

From the 1990s, the more neoliberal approach and greater managerialism in the health care system has seen 'community care' increasingly coming to mean provision of care by a variety of agencies and individuals. These include NHS staff, local authority social services or housing departments, voluntary sector agencies, private institutions such as care homes as well as unpaid informal carers (Cooke and Philpin, 2008). The move to community care showed recognition of the criticisms made of institutional living. However, it also reflected concerns to cut costs and involve 'consumers' in the business of health, especially the families of people who are chronically ill or disabled. In the 1990s 'partnership' was promoted as a way to promote good working between different health and social care agencies but it was also described as a way to involve communities and individuals in how care is planned and provided.

Not surprisingly then, community care has complicated implications for health care 'consumers'. Lindsay Prior, writing in 1993, noted that for some people, life in the community might not be all that different from living in an institution. In addition, much of the care work that goes on in our society is carried out by people who are not paid to do it. Most are family members, usually women. Today, the reduction of welfare has resulted in an international crisis of care (Razavi, 2011). In Britain as many as three million people (one person in every eight) perform paid work as well as unpaid care (Carers UK, cited in Tomkins and Eatough, 2012: 2).

Participation

In all parts of Britain, improving accountability is also linked to a shift towards 'patient-centred' care. Attempts have been made to institutionalize a shift away from paternalism towards a system which 'empowers' people to take responsibility for their own health. Where medical professionals had been likened in the past to modern priests, it has been suggested that today they should change 'from priest to mountain guide' (Hilton, 2008), a metaphor which implies a very different relationship with service users (Cowden and Singh, 2007). However, it has been suggested that the argument that patients will be empowered if they take more responsibility for their own health may be just another way of avoiding the cost of care (Cooke, 2002). 'Empowerment' may work to reinforce existing power imbalances, rather than challenge them (Powers, 2003). The idea that the role of government is to 'nudge' individuals to change health-related behaviours, for example, has been criticized by the British Medical Association, who argue this approach distracts attention from factors outside of the control of individuals (BMA, 2012).

Globalization and Health

The policy changes described above are specific to Britain but also reflect a wider context. The move towards more market-driven approaches to health has been occurring over several decades worldwide, as has the profound shift in power between health professionals and managers (Jarman and Greer, 2010b). This highlights Britain's interconnection with a world that is becoming increasingly globalized.

> Globalization: a process of increasing global economic and cultural inter-connection between localities, nations and regions which involves the exchange of finance, people, products and information.

Whilst different parts of the world have been connected through long distance trade routes for centuries, nineteenth-century industrialization led to the development of a world economy whose fate had implications for all countries. The interconnectedness of our global world accelerated in the twentieth century, with further internationalization of money markets, increased migration, the rise of new transnational political alliances and increased international contact through electronic communication. Though most people in the world still live and work in the same place, human beings are more mobile than ever before, both in terms of where we live and also where we work (Urry, 2007). Issues of global concern have become part of everyday local life (Beck, 2002: 17).

Globalization has a multitude of health implications. For example, whilst it is still the case that most people in the world cannot afford to travel far during their lives (Brubaker, 2005), globalization is associated with new movements of people. British health professionals are increasingly actively recruited from the majority world. Health care is commodified, with international private companies producing services, equipment and health insurance (Jarman and Greer, 2010b). International movements of people also bring new risks of distribution of pathogens, for example, the spread of infection during air travel and of STDs through sex tourism (Ritzer, 2010). New international alignments brought about by globalization mean health policy is decided at levels higher than the nation, for example, the European Union (Greer and Kurzer, 2013).

Another consequence of globalization is medical tourism, with people who can afford to increasingly travelling overseas to obtain the care they need (Hall, 2011). One more sinister development is the growing trade in body parts, legal and illegal, usually from the majority world to the developed world. Perhaps 5–10% of transplanted kidneys, for example, have been purchased, not donated (Epstein, 2009). The rise of human trafficking including sex trafficking also has serious but under-researched health implications (Zimmerman and Stöckl, 2012). Whilst globalization is credited with opening borders, it has also provoked new fears leading to greater regulation of migration and discrimination against refugees worldwide, reflected in the poor health of asylum seekers in Britain (see Chapter 4).

The background to all of these problems is changes in prosperity. Whilst the living standards of some people in countries like China is increasing, the monopolization of food production by a small number of companies and global shifts in control of access to land, fish, animals, plants and water all impact negatively on the global poor. As our climate changes, perhaps catastrophically, it is the poorest in society who will be affected first by heat waves and other extreme events, changes in patterns of infectious disease, changed food yields and freshwater supplies, damaged ecosystems, and displacement and loss of livelihood (McMichael et al., 2008: 191/2).

Nonetheless, globalization also offers new opportunities for people to share knowledge and experience. **Lay epidemiology** and the global environmental justice movement, for example, are approaches to health that can be seen worldwide which reject the framing of community health problems as individual problems. These approaches involve the linking of local campaigns to require industrial, national and international bodies to take responsibility for negative health consequences of production decisions. They demand openness and accountability in the use of scientific and technological expertise, and the right for local people to be involved in decisions that have implications for their health. These movements reflect a global context where many people are well-informed and seek active involvement in health care decisions (Brown, 1992; Kramnaimuang et al., 2012).

Lay epidemiology: the process by which lay people, incorporating information from various agencies, come to their own understanding of health risks and reasons behind the distribution of disease in human populations.

Implications for Practice

The growth of interprofessional practice puts pressure on health and social care professions to find commonalities of practice but also to defend or adapt skills which have been considered key to each profession. This is occurring in a global neoliberal context which threatens both health care resources and living standards, with implications for the amount and the nature of health care work. Concerns about accountability mean that the amount of bureaucracy and the demands of managers for change are also unlikely to lessen. These factors provide the parameters in which the everyday work of health care teams and individual professionals will be carried out. However, it is also important to remember that these parameters have been subject to change and will continue to change, and that health care professionals and service users themselves have been and will increasingly be key actors shaping those changes.

Summary

- Since their inception, health care professionals have actively worked to promote their professions and to shape the particular roles they play in British health and social care systems

- The challenges they face in doing this reflect governmental and manage-rial attempts to shape these systems in particular ways in the context of wider global social, political and economic forces
- The understandings, expectations and demands of health care profes-sionals, increasingly alongside service users, are also important features of the ever-changing global health environment

Exercise

How do you think health policy might change over the next century? How might the work of health professionals change? How do you think they should change?

Further Reading

To learn more about the history of changes to the NHS, use the Nuffield Trust interactive timeline at: http://nhstimeline.nuffieldtrust.org.uk/

Alaszewski, A. and Brown, P. (2012) *Making Health Policy: A Critical Introduction.* Cambridge: Polity.

Ham, C. (2009) *Health Policy in Britain.* Sixth edition. London: Palgrave Macmillan.

Klein, R. (2010) *The New Politics of the NHS. From Creation to Reinvention.* Abingdon, Oxon: Radcliffe.

 Online readings

To access further resources related to this chapter, visit the companion web-site at www.sagepub.co.uk/russell

Cowden, S. and Singh, Gurnam (2007) 'The "user": friend, foe or fetish? A criti-cal exploration of user involvement in health and social care', *Critical Social Policy* 27(1): 5–23.

Glossary

Ageism – discrimination based on a person's age

Barrier – a physical, social or economic obstacle that prevents the equal participation of disabled people in society

Biographical disruption – occurs when a person is forced to re-think who they are and where their life is going (their biography) as a result of being diagnosed with a chronic illness

Biomedicine, biomedical model – an approach to health and illness which defines illness as the absence of disease, portraying the human organism as either functioning 'normally' or else dysfunctional and therefore diseased

Biopsychosocial model – an approach to health and illness which sees illness as reflecting psychological and social as well as biological factors

Bureaucracy – the hierarchical administration of an organization by a body of non-elected officials

Capitalism – a society in which ownership and control of production and business for profit in a competitive economy is the most important means of access to wealth and power

Class – see social class

Cohort – a group of people who share a significant event or experience in a specified time, for example, those born in the same year or decade

Cultural resources (or cultural capital) – assets such as knowledge, skills and competencies that a person can use to improve their social position in society

Disablism – discrimination or prejudice against people with disabilities

Discourse – a way of talking about and thinking about something that influences the way we experience it

(The) Enlightenment – an intellectual and cultural movement in Western Europe c1650–1800 which introduced many ideas and ideals associated with modern society

Equality Act 2010 – legislation designed to protect people in Britain from discrimination on the basis of age, disability, gender assignment, marriage and civil partnership, pregnancy and maternity, race, religion or belief, sex or sexual orientation

Ethnic minority – a group of people who have a shared language, culture and way of life that is different from the majority in the society where they live

Ethnicity – an identity that locates a person as belonging to a group who see themselves as distinct on the basis of shared characteristics such as kin, history, heritage, language, religion and nationality

Eugenics movement – the 'science' of controlling human breeding to discourage the birth of people cast as genetically inferior, including disabled and gay people and those from ethnic minority groups

Gender – an aspect of identity that we make when we act or speak in ways that show our sense of what it means to be male or female

Germ theory – an explanation which identified micro-organisms as the essential agent for particular infectious diseases

Globalization – a process of increasing global economic and cultural interconnection between localities, nations and regions which involves the exchange of finance, people, products and information

Hate crime – a criminal offence committed against a person or property motivated by hostility towards someone based on their disability, race, religion, gender identity or sexual orientation

Hegemonic masculinity – the way of 'doing' gender that is most valued in our society (the best people are the ones who can 'be a man')

Heterosexism – the belief that heterosexuality is superior to homosexuality, the assumption that everyone is or should be heterosexual (see Julie Fish definition in Chapter 7)

Iatrogenesis – medical intervention which, instead of curing, actually causes illness

Identity – how we categorize ourselves in relation to others

Infantilization – treating a non-infant as if they were an infant

Institutional racism – where an institution discriminates against ethnic minority people because of ingrained attitudes and practices that work to disadvantage ethnic minority people

Intersex – someone whose sex may be difficult to categorize as male or female due to ambiguous genitalia or other biological characteristics

Labelling – a process whereby a person who receives a diagnosis changes because of the changed reactions of other people to them

Lay epidemiology – the process by which lay people, incorporating information from various agencies, come to their own understanding of health risks and reasons behind the distribution of disease in human populations

Lay person – a person who is not an expert in a particular area

Life course – the sequence of events and activities, reflecting social expectations and institutions, that we encounter as we move from birth through to death

Majority world – a term used in preference to 'developing' or 'third world' countries, which attempts to avoid describing those countries in terms of how they appear from the viewpoint of those in the wealthiest countries

Managerialism – the application of managerial techniques to running non-business organizations like the civil service and local authorities

Masculinities and femininities – ways of speaking and behaving that reflect socially constructed ideas about what it means to be male or female

Mechanical metaphor – a feature of the biomedical model of illness that portrays the human body as functioning essentially like a machine

Medical gaze – refers to the way in which medical professionals offer a view and a vision of how the human body works which comes to be adopted by lay people

Medicalization – a process by which previously non-medical issues in society come to be thought of and understood in a medical way

Neoliberalism – a political approach which favours minimal government intervention in business and reducing spending on welfare

Norms – informal understandings amongst groups of people about the right way to behave

Party – an organization which works to attain material advantages for its members and increase their social power

Personhood – the status of being counted as a person

Power – a capacity to dominate in relation to the actions or ideas of other people

Psychosocial factors – social experiences and environments which cause stress for individuals, making them more vulnerable to illness

Psychosis/psychotic disorders – disorders whose main symptom is impairment of a person's ability to perceive reality, expressed mainly in delusions or hallucinations

Racism – words or actions which reflect a view that human beings can be divided into sub-species, and that some sub-species are superior to others

Reliability – a finding is reliable when you can obtain the same result even when you use different ways of measuring the same thing

Sex – whether a person has the anatomical characteristics normally associated with men or women

Social capital – a resource that can be held by individuals which relates to their connectedness with others

Social class – a grouping of people who share a similar situation in society based on their access to property and other resources

Social construction – a concept used to emphasize the social or cultural rather than biological basis of social divisions and differences

Social control – processes in society that ensure people follow the formal and informal rules of society

Social determinants of health – the circumstances in which people live that affect their health, including the health system available to them

Social factors – factors which affect an individual and involve other people, including the many people to whose lives we are indirectly connected even though we may never have met them (for example, wider social groups to which we are connected such as our class, gender, ethnic group, sexuality and nation)

Social model of disability – emphasizes that disability occurs when society fails to take the necessary steps to facilitate full participation of people who have impairments

Socio-economic status – a measure of social position which takes into account income, education and occupation

Sociology – the systematic study of human beings in society

The state/states – the government and national institutions they control that are paid for through taxation including the civil service, legal system, schools and universities

Status – honour or prestige acquired by different social groups in society that increases their social power

Surveillance – refers to the close monitoring of a group of people which may influence their behaviour

Transgender – someone who does not easily fit into the social norm whereby people are seen as being born either male or female and as having particular desires, personalities and behaviours biologically fixed by their sex

Urbanicity – the impact of living in an urban area at a given time, taking into account that there may be degrees to which an environment can be described as urban depending on factors such as population density

Key theorists and the concepts with which they are associated

Peter Blau	dynamics of bureaucracy
Michael Bury	biographical disruption
Kathy Charmaz	loss of self
Raewyn Connell	hegemonic masculinity
René Descartes	mind/body dualism
Norbert Elias	the civilizing process
George Engel	the biopsychosocial model
Michel Foucault	the medical gaze; discourse; surveillance
Eliot Friedson	professional dominance
Erving Goffman	stigma; asylums
Arlie Hochschild	emotional labour
Ivan Illich	iatrogenesis
Allison James and Alan Prout	the new sociology of childhood
Terry Johnson	professional power
Peter Laslett	the third age
Michael Marmot, Richard Wilkinson	psychosocial factors, social determinants of health
Karl Marx, Friedrich Engels	capitalism
Sarah Nettleton	the mechanical metaphor
Ann Oakley	the medicalization of childbirth

Talcott Parsons	the sick role
Graham Scambler	felt and enacted stigma
Thomas Scheff	labelling theory
Thomas Szasz	the myth of mental illness; labelling
Peter Townsend	relative and absolute poverty; structured dependency
Max Weber	class, status and party; bureaucracy and the 'iron cage'
Anne Witz	professions and patriarchy
Irving Zola	medicalization

References

Abel, T. and Frohlich, K. (2012) 'Capitals and capabilities: linking structure and agency to reduce health inequalities', *Social Science and Medicine*, 74(2): 236–44.

Addis, S., Davies, M., Greene, G., MacBride-Stewart, S. and Shepherd, M. (2009) 'The health, social care and housing needs of lesbian, gay, bisexual and transgender older people: a review of the literature', *Health and Social Care in the Community*, 17(6): 647–58.

Afifi, M. (2007) 'Gender differences in mental health', *Singapore Medical Journal*, 48(5): 385–91.

Age Concern (2007) *Final Report, UK Inquiry into Mental Health and Well-being in Later Life*. London: Age Concern.

Agius, S. and Tobler, C. (2012) *Trans and Intersex People. Discrimination on the Grounds of Sex, Gender Identity and Gender Expression*. European Network of Legal Experts in the Non-Discrimination Field. Luxembourg: European Union.

Ahmad, W. and Bradby, H. (eds) (2009) *Ethnicity, Health and Health Care. Understanding Diversity, Tacking Disadvantage*. Malden/Oxford: Blackwell.

Ahmad, W.I.U., Atkin, K. and Chamba, R. (2000) '"Causing havoc to their children": parental and professional perspectives on consanguinity and childhood disability', in W.I.U. Ahmad (ed.) *Ethnicity, Disability and Chronic Illness*. Buckingham: Open University Press, 28–44.

Albanese, E., Banerjee, S., Dhanasiri, S., Fernandez, J., Ferri, C., Knapp, M., McCrone, P., Prince, M., Snell, T. and Stewart, R. (2007) *Dementia UK. Summary of Key Findings*. London: Alzheimer's Society.

Alemany, S., Goldberg, X., van Winkel, R., Gastó, C. and Fañanás, L. (2012) 'Childhood adversity and psychosis: examining whether the association is due to genetic confounding using a monozygotic twin differences approach', *European Psychiatry*, doi:10.1016/j.eurpsy.2012.03.001.

Annandale, E. (2009) *Women's Health and Social Change*. London: Routledge.

Annandale, E. and Field, K. (2007) 'Gender differences in health', in S. Taylor and D. Field (eds) (2007) *Sociology of Health and Health Care*. Oxford: Blackwell, 93–112.

Annandale, E. and Riska, E. (2009) 'New connections: towards a gender-inclusive approach to women's and men's health', *Current Sociology*, 57: 123–33.

Atkinson, D. and Walmsley, J. (2010) 'History from the inside: towards an inclusive history of intellectual disability', *Scandinavian Journal of Disability Research*, 12(4): 273–86.

Atkinson, P. (1988) 'Discourse, descriptions and diagnosis: reproducing normal medicine', in M. Lock and D. Gordon (eds) *Biomedicine Examined*. London: Kluwer Academic Publishers, 179–204.

Bagwell, C E. (2005) '"Respectful Image". Revenge of the Barber Surgeon', *Annals of Surgery*, 241(6): 872–78.

Barford, A., Dorling, D., Davey-Smith, G. and Shaw, M. (2006) 'Life expectancy: women now on top everywhere', *British Medical Journal*, 332: 808.

Barker, M., Richards, C., Jones, R., Bowes-Catton, H. and Plowman, T. (of BiUK) with Yockney, J. (of Bi Community News) and Morgan, M. (of The Bisexual Index) (2012) *The Bisexuality Report: Bisexual Inclusion in LGBT Equality and Diversity*. Centre for Citizenship, Identities and Governance and Faculty of Health and Social Care. Maidenhead: Open University.

Barnes, C. and Mercer, G. (2010) *Exploring Disability: A Sociological Introduction*. Second Edition. Cambridge: Polity.

Barr, B., Taylor-Robinson, D., Scott-Samuel, A., McKee, M. and Stuckler, D. et al. (2012) 'Suicides associated with the 2008–10 economic recession in England: time trend analysis', *British Medical Journal*, 345: e5142.

Bartley, M. and Blane, D. (2009) 'Life-course influences on health at later ages', in H. Graham (ed.) *Understanding Health Inequalities*. Second edition. Maidenhead: Open University Press, McGraw-Hill Education, 48–65.

Bartley, M., Popay, J. and Plewis, I. (1992) 'Domestic conditions, paid employment and women's experiences of ill-health', *Sociology of Health and Illness*, 14(3): 313–43.

Bashford, A. and Levine, P. (2010) *The Oxford Handbook of the History of Eugenics*. Oxford: Oxford University Press.

Bécares, L. (2009) *The Ethnic Density Effect on the Health of Ethnic Minority People in the United Kingdom: A Study of Hypothesised Pathways*. PhD dissertation, University College London.

Bécares, L. and Das-Munshi, J. (2013) 'Ethnic density, health care seeking behaviour and expected discrimination from health services among ethnic minority people in England', *Health and Place*, July, 22: 48–55.

Beck, U. (1992) *Risk Society: Towards a New Modernity*. London: Sage.

Beck, U. (2002) 'The cosmopolitan society and its enemies', *Theory, Culture and Society*, 19(1–2): 17–44.

Becker, C.M., Glascoff, M.A. and Felts, W.M. (2010) 'Salutogenesis 30 years later: where do we go from here?' *International Electronic Journal of Health Education*, 13: 25–32.

Benatar, S.R., Gill, S. and Bakker, I. (2011) 'Global health and the global economic crisis', *American Journal of Public Health*, 101(4): 646–53.

Benedict, R. (1943) *Race and Racism*. London: Routledge and Kegan Paul.

Bennett, D. (2012) 'Elder abuse and death claims', *The AvMA Medical and Legal Journal*, 18(5): 194.

Bentley, K. (2005) 'Women, mental health, and the psychiatric enterprise: a review', *Health and Social Work*, 30(1): 56–63.

Bhugra, D. (2004) 'Migration and mental health', *Acta Psychiatrica Scandinvavia*, 109(4): 243–58.

Blaise, M. (2005) *Playing it Straight: Uncovering Gender Discourse in the Early Childhood*. London: Routledge.

Blau, P.M. (1963) *The Dynamics of Bureaucracy: A Study of Interpersonal Relations in Two Government Agencies*. Second Edition. Chicago: University of Chicago Press.

Bloch, A. and Solomos, J. (eds) (2009) *Race and Ethnicity in the Twenty-First Century*. Basingstoke, New York: Palgrave Macmillan.

Blume, S. (2010) *The Artificial Ear: Cochlear Implants and the Culture of Deafness*. New Brunswick, N.J.: Rutgers University Press.

Bond, J., Peace, S.M., Dittmann-Kohli, F. and Westerhof, G. (2007) *Ageing in Society: An Introduction to Social Gerontology*. Third edition. London: Sage.

Bourdieu, P. (1991) *Language and Symbolic Power*. Cambridge: Polity.

Bowling, A. and Cartwright, A. (1982) *Life After Death: A Study of Elderly Widowed*. London: Tavistock.

Bradby, H. (2008) 'Editorial: Virtual Special Issue on Feminism and the Sociology of Gender, Health and Illness', *Sociology of Health and Illness*.

Braverman, P. (2009) 'Health disparities beginning in childhood: a life-course perspective', *Pediatrics*, 124: S163–S175.

British Medical Association (BMA) (2012) Behaviour Change, Public Health and the Role of the State – BMA Position Statement. London: BMA.

Brown, G.W. (1989) 'Life events and measurement', in G.W. Brown and T.O. Harris (eds) *Life Events and Illness*. London: The Guildford Press, 3–48.

Brown, I. and Brown, R.I. (2003) *Quality of Life and Disability. An Approach for Community Practitioners*. London: Jessica Kingsley.

Brown, P. (1992) 'Popular epidemiology and toxic waste contamination: lay and professional ways of knowing', *Journal of Health and Social Behavior*, 33: 267–81.

Brubaker, R. (2004) *Ethnicity Without Groups*. Harvard: President and Fellows of Harvard College.

Brubaker, R. (2005) 'The "Diaspora" diaspora', *Ethnic and Racial Studies* 28(1): 1–19.

Bruinius, H. (2007) *Better for All the World. The Secret History of Forced Sterilization and America's Quest for Racial Purity*. New York: Vintage.

Brunton, D. (ed.) (2004) *Medicine Transformed: Health, Disease and Society in Europe 1800–1930*. Manchester: Manchester University Press.

Bury, M. (1982) 'Chronic illness as biographical disruption', *Sociology of Health and Illness*, 4(2): 167–82.

Byard, W. and Krous, H.F. (2003) 'Sudden Infant Death Syndrome: overview and update', *Pediatric and Developmental Pathology*, 6(2): 112–27.

Cacchioni, T. And Tiefer, L. (2012) 'Why medicalization? Introduction on the special issue on the medicalization of sex', *Journal of Sex Research*, 49(4): 307–10.

Cantor-Graae, E. and Selten, J.P. (2005) 'Schizophrenia and migration: a meta-analysis and review', *American Journal of Psychiatry*, 162(1): 12–24.

Carter, R. (2007) Genes, Genomes and Genealogies: The Return of Scientific Racism. *Ethnic and Racial Studies* 30(4): 546–556.

Caulfield, T., Ries, N.M., Ray, P.N., Shuman, C. and Wilson, B.(2010) 'Direct-to-consumer genetic testing: good, bad or benign?' *Clinical Genetics*, 77: 101–05.

Charmaz, K. (1983) 'Loss of self: a fundamental form of suffering in the chronically ill', *Sociology of Health and Illness*, 5(2): 168–95.

Charmaz, K. (1991) *Good Days, Bad Days: The Self in Chronic Illness and Time.* New Jersey: Rutgers University Press.

Charmaz, K. (2000) 'Experiencing chronic illness', in G.L. Albrecht, R. Fitzpatrick and S.C. Scrimshaw (eds) *The Handbook of Social Studies in Health and Medicine.* London: Sage, 277–92.

Chaturvedi, N. (2003) 'Ethnic differences in cardiovascular disease', *Heart,* 89(6): 681–6.

Chinn, D. (2011) 'Critical health literacy: a review and critical analysis', *Social Science and Medicine,* 73(1): 60–7.

Connell, R.W. and Messerschmidt, J.W. (2005) 'Hegemonic masculinity: rethinking the concept', *Gender and Society,* 19(6): 829–59.

Conrad, P. and Angell, A. (2004) 'Homosexuality and remedicalization', *Society,* 41(5): 32–9.

Cooke, H. (2002) 'Empowerment', in G. Blakely and V. Bryson (eds) *Contemporary Political Concepts.* London: Pluto, 162–78.

Cooke, H. and Philpin, S. (2008) *Sociology in Nursing and Health Care.* Edinburgh: Elsevier.

Corr, S., Petchesky, R. and Parker, R. (2008) *Sexuality, Health and Human Rights.* London: Routledge.

Cort, E. et al. (2004) 'Couples in palliative care', *Sexual and Relationship Therapy,* 19(3): 337–54.

Cottingham, J. and Berer, M. (2011) 'Access to essential medicines for sexual and reproductive health care: the role of the pharmaceutical industry and international regulation', *Reproductive Health Matters,* 19(38): 69–84.

Courtenay, W.H. (2000) 'Constructions of masculinity and their influence on men's well-being: a theory of gender and health', *Social Science and Medicine,* 50: 1385–401.

Cowden, S. and Singh, G. (2007) 'The "user": friend, foe or fetish? A critical exploration of user involvement in health and social care', *Critical Social Policy,* 27(1): 5–23.

Craig, T.K.J. (2011) 'Chapter 8: Psychosis, migration and ethnic minority status: a story of inequality, rejection and discrimination', in D. Bhugra and S. Gupta (eds) *Migration and Mental Health.* Cambridge: Cambridge University Press: 107–116.

Crawford, R. (2008) 'The politics of victim blaming', in S. Earle and G. Letherby (eds) *The Sociology of Healthcare. A Reader for Health Professionals.* Basingstoke: Palgrave MacMillan: 123–35.

Creighton, G. and Oliffe, J.L. (2010) 'Theorising masculinities and men's health: a brief history with a view to practice', *Health Sociology Review,* 19: 409–18.

Cribb, J., Joyce, R. and Philip, D. (2012) *Living Standards, Poverty and Inequality in the UK: 2012.* London: Institute for Fiscal Studies, Joseph Rowntree Foundation.

Cumming, E. and Henry, W.E. (1961) *Growing Old: The Process of Disengagement.* New York: Basic.

Darr, A., Astin, K. and Atkin, K. (2008) 'Causal Attributions, lifestyle change and coronary heart disease: illness beliefs of patients of South Asian and European origin living in the UK', *Heart and Lung – The Journal of Acute and Critical Care*, 37(2): 91–104.

Das-Munshi, J., Clark, C., Dewey, M.E., Leavey, G., Stansfeld, S.A. and Prince, M.J. (2013) 'Does childhood adversity account for poorer mental and physical health in second-generation Irish people living in Britain? Birth cohort study from Britain (NCDS)', *British Medical Journal Open*, 3: 1–10.

Davey Smith, G. (2000) 'Learning to live with complexity: ethnicity, socioeconomic position, and health in Britain and the United States', *American Journal of Public Health*, 90(11): 1694–98.

Davies, C. (1995) *Gender and the Professional Predicament in Nursing*. Buckingham: Open University Press.

Davies, J. and Davies, D. (2010) 'Origins and evolution of antibiotic resistance', *Microbiology and Molecular Biology Reviews*, 74(3): 417–33.

Davies, J.B., Sandstrom, S., Shorrocks, A. and Wolff, E.N. (2008) *The World Distribution of Household Wealth*. New York: World Institute for Development Economics Research of the United Nations.

Davis, A. and George, J. (1993) *States of Health: Health and Illness in Australia*. Second Edition. Melbourne: Longman.

De Bont, R. (2010) 'Schizophrenia, evolution and the borders of biology: on Huxley et al.'s 1964 paper in Nature', *History of Psychiatry*, 21: 144–59.

Deacon, H. and Stephney, I. (2007) *HIV/AIDS, Stigma and Children: A Literature Review*. Capetown: Human Sciences Research Council.

Department for Work and Pensions (2011) *The Pensioners' Incomes Series 2010–11*. London: The Stationery Office.

Department of Health (DoH) (2009) *Tackling Health Inequalities: 10 Years On. A Review of Developments in Tackling Health Inequalities in England over the Last 10 Years*. London: Department of Health.

Dorling, D. (2012) 'Inequality constitutes a particular place', *Social and Cultural Geography*, 13(1): 1–10.

Dorling, D. (2013) *Unequal Health: The Scandal of Our Times*. Bristol: Policy Press.

Doyal, L. (1995) *What Makes Women Sick: Gender and the Political Economy of Health*. London: Macmillan.

Dunstan, S. (ed.) (2012) *General Lifestyle Survey Overview*. London: ONS.

Dyson, S.M. and Atkin, K. (2011) 'Sickle cell and Thalassaemia: global public health issues come of age', *Ethnicity and Health*, 16(4–5): 299–311.

Earle, S. (2003) 'Disability and stigma: an unequal life', *Speech and Language Therapy in Practice*, 1–12.

Edwards, J. (2012) 'The healthcare needs of gay and lesbian patients', in E. Kuhlman and E. Annandale (eds) *The Palgrave Handbook of Gender and Healthcare*. Palgrave Macmillan: 290–305.

Eichler, K., Wieser, S. and Brügger, U. (2009) 'The costs of limited health literacy: a systematic review', *International Journal of Public Health*, 54: 313–24.

Elias, N. (2000) *The Civilizing Process: Sociogenetic and Psychogenetic Investigations*. Revised edition. Oxford: Blackwell.

Elmer, P. (ed.) (2004) *The Healing Arts: Health, Disease and Society in Europe, 1500–1800*. Manchester: Manchester University Press.

Elmslie, C. and Hunt, K. (2009) 'Men, masculinities and heart disease: a systematic review of the qualitative literature', *Current Sociology,* 57: 155–91.

Emerson, E., Baines, S., Allerton, L. and Welch, V. (2012) *Health Inequalities and People with Learning Disabilities in the UK: 2012*. Improving Health and Lives: Learning Disabilities Observatory. London: Department of Health.

Engel, G. L. (1977) 'The need for a new medical model: a challenge for biomedicine', *Science*, 196, 2486, 8 April: 129–36.

Engels, F. (1845/2006) *The Condition of the Working Class in England in 1844*. Revised edition. London: Penguin.

Engelhardt, H.T. (1981) 'The disease of masturbation: values and the concept of disease', in A. Caplan, H.T. Engelhardt and J.J. McCartney (eds) *Concepts of Health and Disease*. Reading, MA: Addison-Wesley.

Epstein, M. (2009) Sociological and ethical issues in transplant commercialism. *Current Opinion in Organ Transplantation* 14(2): 134–39.

Evans, O., Singelton, N., Meltzer, H., Stewart, R. and Prince, M. (2003) *The Mental Health of Older People*. London: HMSO.

Evans-Lacko, S., Henderson, C. and Thornicroft, G. (2013) 'Public knowledge, attitudes and behaviour regarding people with mental illness in England 2009–2012', *British Journal of Psychiatry*, 202: s51–s57.

Felde, L.H. (2011) 'Elevated Cholesterol as Biographical Work – Expanding the Concept of "Biographical Disruption"', *Qualitative Sociology Review* 7(2): 101–20.

Fernando, S. (2010) 'DSM-5 and the "Psychosis Risk Syndrome"', *Psychosis: Psychological, Social and Integrative Approaches*, 2(3): 196–98.

Field, D. and Kelly, M.P. (2007) 'Chronic illness and physical disability', in S. Taylor and D. Field (eds) *Sociology of Health and Health Care*. Oxford: Blackwell, 137–58.

Fish, J. (2010) 'Promoting equality and valuing diversity for lesbian, gay, bisexual and trans patients', *InnovAiT,* 3(6): 333–8.

Fish, J. and Hunt, R. (2008) *Prescription for Change. Lesbian and Bisexual Women's Health Check*. London: Stonewall.

Fitzpatrick, R. (2008) 'Chapter One: Society and changing patterns of disease', in G. Scambler (ed.) *Sociology as Applied to Medicine*. Sixth edition. London: W. B. Saunders, 3–17.

Fortier, A. (2011) 'Genetic indigenisation in "The People of the British Isles"', *Science as Culture*, 21(2): 153–75.

Foucault, M. (1965) *Madness and Civilization: A History of Insanity in the Age of Reason*. New York: Pantheon.

Foucault, M. (1975) *Discipline and Punish. The Birth of the Prison*. New York: Random House.

Foucault, M. (1977) *Discipline and Punish*. Harmondsworth: Penguin.

Foucault, M. (1978) *The History of Sexuality. Volume 1*. New York: Pantheon.

Frank, A.W. (1995) *The Wounded Storyteller: Body, Illness and Ethics*. Chicago: University of Chicago Press.

Friedson, E. (1975) *Profession of Medicine. A Study of the Sociology of Applied Knowledge.* New York: Dodd Mead.

Gabe, J. and Calnan, M. (eds) (2009) *The New Sociology of the Health Service.* Oxon, New York: Routledge.

Gabe, J., Bury, M. and Elston, M.A. (2004) *Key Concepts in Medical Sociology.* London: Sage.

Gabe, J., Kelleher, D. and Williams, G. (1994) *Challenging Medicine.* London: Routledge.

Gale, E.A.M. (2002) 'The rise of childhood type 1 diabetes in the 20th century', *Diabetes,* 51, December: 3353–61.

Garrett, C., Gask, L.L., Hays, R., Cherrington, A., Bundy, C., Dickens, C., Waheed, W. and Coventry, P.A. (2012) 'Accessing primary health care: a meta-ethnography of the experiences of British South Asian Patients with diabetes, coronary heart disease or a mental health problem', *Chronic Illness* 8(2): 135–55.

Gilleard, C. and Higgs, P. (2000) *Cultures of Ageing: Self, Citizen and the Body.* Harlow: Prentice Hall.

Gilleard, C. and Higgs, P. (2002) 'The third age: class, cohort or generation?' *Ageing and Society,* 22(3), May: 369–82.

Gilleard, C. and Higgs, P. (2010) 'Frailty, disability and old age: a re-appraisal', *Health,* 15(5): 475–490.

Gjonça, A., Tomassini, B.T. and Smallwood, S. (2005) 'Sex differences in mortality, a comparison of the United Kingdom and other developed countries', *Health Statistics Quarterly,* 26: 6–16.

Goffman, E. (1961) *Asylums. Essays on the Social Situation of Mental Patients and Other Inmates.* New York: Doubleday Anchor.

Goffman, E. (1963) *Stigma: Notes on the Management of Spoiled Identity.* New York: Simon and Schuster.

Gott, M., Galena, E., Hinchliff, S. and Elford, H. (2004) '"Opening a can of worms": GP and practice nurse barriers to talking about sexual health in primary care', *Family Practice,* 21(5): 528–36.

Gottlieb, A. (2004) *The Afterlife is Where We Come From: The Culture of Infancy in West Africa.* Chicago: University of Chicago Press.

Gramsci, A. (1971) *The Prison Notebooks.* London: Lawrence and Wishart.

Green, G., Bradby, H., Chan, A. and Lee, M. (2006) '"We are not completely Westernized": Dual medical systems and pathways to health care among Chinese migrant women in England', *Social Science and Medicine,* 62(6): 1498–509.

Greer, S.L. and Kurzer, P. (eds) (2013) *European Union Public Health Policy: Regional and Global Trends.* London: Routledge.

Griffin, J. and Berry, E.M. (2003) 'A modern day holy anorexia? Religious language in advertising and anorexia nervosa in the West', *European Journal of Clinical Nutrition,* 57: 43–51.

GRO Scotland (2011) *Alcohol-related deaths in Scotland, 1979 to 2011* (web only): www.gro-scotland.gov.uk/statistics/theme/vital-events/deaths/alcohol-related/index.html

Gruen, E. (2011) *Rethinking the Other in Antiquity. Martin Classical Lectures.* Princeton: Princeton University Press.

Grzywacz, J.G., Almeida, D.M., Neupert, S.D. and Ettner, S.L. (2004) 'Socioeconomic status and health: a micro-level analysis of exposure and vulnerability to daily stressors', *Journal of Health and Social Behavior*, 45(1): 1–16.

Haboubi, N.H.J. and Lincoln, N. (2003) 'Views of health professionals on discussing sexual issues with patients', *Disability and Rehabilitation*, 25(6): 291–6.

Hall, M.C. (2011) 'Health and medical tourism? A kill or cure for global public health?' *Tourism Review*, 66(1–2): 4–15.

Hall, S. (1996) 'The West and the rest: discourse and power', in S. Hall, D. Held, D. Hubert and K. Thompson (eds) *Modernity: an Introduction to Modern Societies*. Malden, Oxford, Carlton: Blackwell: 184–227.

Harding, S. (2004) 'Mortality of migrants from the Caribbean to England and Wales: effect of duration of residence', *International Journal of Epidemiology*, 33(2): 382–6.

Hart, N. (1985) 'The sociology of health and medicine', in M. Haralambos (ed.) *Sociology: New Directions*. Orsmkirk: Causeway.

Health and Safety Executive (2012) *The Burden of Occupational Cancer in Great Britain. Overview Report*. London: HSE.

Health Protection Agency (2006) *Migrant Health: Infectious Diseases in Non-UK Born Populations in England, Wales and Northern Ireland. A Baseline Report*. London: HPA.

Healy, D. (2008) *Mania: A Short History of Bipolar Disorder*. Volume 3 of the John Hopkins Biographies of Disease Series. Baltimore, MD: The John Hopkins University Press.

Heath, H. (2002) 'Sexuality and later life', in H. Heath and I. White (eds) *The Challenge of Sexuality in Health Care*. Oxford: Blackwell, 133–52.

Hepp, U., Spindler, A. and Milos, G. (2005) 'Eating disorder symptomatology and gender role orientation', *International Journal of Eating Disorders*, April, 37: 227–33.

Herdt, G. (2004) *The Sambia: Ritual, Sexuality and Change in Papua New Guinea (Case Studies in Cultural Anthropology)*. Belmont, CA: Wadsworth.

Higgs, P. (2008) 'Later life, health and society', in G. Scambler (ed.) *Sociology as Applied to Medicine*. Sixth edition. London: W.B. Saunders.

Hilton, S. (2008) 'Education and the changing face of medical professionalism: from priest to mountain guide?' *The British Journal of General Practice*, 58(550): 353–61.

Hindley, C. and Thomson, A.M. (2005) 'The rhetoric of informed choice: perspectives from midwives on intrapartum fetal heart rate monitoring', *Health Expectations*, 8(4): 306–14.

Hinshaw, S.P. (2005) 'The stigmatization of mental illness in children and parents: developmental issues, family concerns, and research needs', *The Journal of Child Psychology and Psychiatry*, 46(7): 714–34.

Hochschild, A. (1983) *The Managed Heart: The Commercialization of Human Feeling*. Berkeley, CA: University of California Press.

Hockey, J. and James, A. (1993) *Growing up and Growing Old: Ageing and Dependency in the Life Course*. London: Sage.

Holmes, T.H. and Rahe, R.H. (1967) 'The social readjustment rating scale', *Journal of Psychomatic Research,* 11: 213–18.

Horwitz, A. (2002) *Creating Mental Illness.* Chicago: University of Chicago Press.

Howe, L.D, Tilling, K., Galobardes, B., Smith, G.D., Ness, A.R. and Lawlor, D.A. (2011) 'Socioeconomic disparities in trajectories of adiposity across childhood', *International Journal of Pediatric Obesity,* June 6(2–2): e144–53.

Hsu, M.C., Moyle, W., Creedy, D. and Venturato, L. (2005) 'An investigation of aged care mental health knowledge of Queensland aged care nurses', *International Journal of Mental Health Nursing,* March, 14(1): 16–23.

Hughes, B. (2000) 'Medicalized bodies', in P. Hancock, B. Hughes, E. Jagger, K. Paterson, R. Russell, E. Tulle-Winton and M. Tyler, *The Body, Culture and Society: An Introduction.* Buckingham: Open University Press, 12–28.

Hughes, B. and Paterson, K. (1997) 'The social model of disability and the disappearing body: towards a sociology of impairment', *Disability and Society,* 12(3): 325–40.

Hughes, K., Bellis, M.A., Jones, L., Wood, S., Bates, G., Eckley, L., McCoy, E., Mikton, C., Shakespeare, T. and Officer, A. (2012) 'Prevalence and risk of violence against adults with disabilities: a systematic review and meta-analysis of observational studies', *Lancet,* Published online. doi:10.1016/S0410-6736(11)61851-5.

Hunt, K., Hannah, M.K. and West, P. (2004) 'Contextualising smoking: masculinity, femininity and class differences in smoking in men and women from three generations in the west of Scotland', *Health Education Research,* June, 19(3): 239–49.

Hunt, K. and Batty, D.G. (2009) 'Gender and socio-economic inequalities in mortality and health behaviours: an overview', in H. Graham, *Understanding Health Inequalities.* Second edition. Maidenhead: OUP, McGraw Hill, 141–61.

Hurcombe, R., Bayley, M. and Goodman, A. (2010) *Ethnicity and Alcohol: A Review of the UK Literature.* York: Joseph Rowntree Foundation.

Hutchison, E.D. (2011) 'Chapter One: A life course perspective', in E.D. Hutchison (ed.) *Dimensions of Human Behavior. The Changing Life Course.* Fourth edition. Thousand Oaks, CA: Sage, 1–38.

Illich, I. (1976) *Limits to Medicine. Medical Nemesis: The Appropriation of Health.* London: Marion Boyars.

International Telecommunications Union (ITU) Broadband Commission for Digital Development (2012) *The State of Broadband 2012: Achieving Digital Inclusion for All.* New York: Broadband Commission.

IPPR (2012) 'Eight out of Ten Married Women do more Housework than their Husbands'. Press release, 10 March 2012. Available at: www.ippr.org/press-releases/111/8831/eight-out-of-ten-married-women-do-more-housework-than-their-husbands

James, A. and Prout, A. (2005) *Constructing and Reconstructing Childhood. Contemporary Issues in the Sociological Study of Childhood.* Second edition. London: Falmer Press.

Jarman, H. and Greer, S.L. (2010a) 'In the eye of the storm: civil servants and managers in the UK Department of Health', *Social Policy and Administration,* 44(2): 172–92.

Jarman, H. and Greer, S.L. (2010b) 'Crossborder trade in health services: lessons from the European Laboratory', *Health Policy*, 94(2): 158–63.

Jarvis, G.E. (2008) 'Changing psychiatric perception of African Americans with psychosis', *European Journal of American Culture*, 27(3): 227–52.

Jayaweera, H. (2010) *Health and Access to Health Care of Migrants in the UK*. A Race Equality Foundation Briefing Paper. Better Health Briefing 19.

Jewson, N. (1976) 'The disappearance of the sick man from medical cosmology 1770–1870', *Sociology*, 10: 225–44.

Johnson, T. (1972) *Professions and Power*. London: Heinemann.

Jones, L., Bellis, M.A., Wood, S., Hughes, K., McCoy, E., Eckley, L, Bates, G., Mikton, C., Shakespeare, T. and Officer, A. (2012) 'Prevalence and risk of violence against children with disabilities: a systematic review and meta-analysis of observational studies', *Lancet*. Published online. doi:10.1016/S0140-6736(12)60692-8.

Joshi, H., Wiggins, R.D., Bartley, M., Mitchell, R., Gleave, S. and Lynch, K. (2008) 'The determinants of geographical inequalities in health', in S. Earle and G. Letherby (eds) *The Sociology of Healthcare. A Reader for Health Professionals*. Basingstoke: Palgrave MacMillan: 136–48.

Kampf, A. and Botelho, L.A. (2009) 'Anti-aging and biomedicine: critical studies on the pursuit of maintaining, revitalizing and enhancing aging bodies', *Medicine Studies*, 1: 187–95.

Karner, Christian (2007) *Ethnicity and Everyday Life*. London: Routledge.

Katz, S. (1996) *Disciplining Old Age: The Formations of Gerontological Knowledge*. Charlottesville, VA: University of Virginia Press.

Kaufman, S.R., Shim, J.K. and Russ, A.J. (2004) 'Revisiting the biomedicalization of aging: clinical trends and ethical challenges', *Gerontologist*, Dec, 44(6), December: 731–7.

Kendig, H. and Browning, C. (2010) 'A social view on healthy ageing: multi-disciplinary perspectives and Australian evidence', in D. Dannefer and C. Phillipson (eds) *The Sage Handbook of Social Gerontology*. London: Sage, 459–71.

Kennedy, P. and Kennedy, C.A. (2010) *Using Theory to Explore Health, Medicine and Society*. Bristol: Policy Press.

King, M., Semlyen, J., See Tai, S., Killaspy, H., Osborn, D., Popelyuk, D. and Nazareth, I. (2008) 'A systematic review of mental disorder, suicide and deliberate self harm in lesbian, gay and bisexual people', *BMC Psychiatry*, 8: 70.

Kirkbride, J.B., Errazuriz, A., Croudace, T.J., Morgan, C., Jackson, D., McCrone, P., Murray, R.M. and Jones, P.B. (2011) 'Systematic Review of the Incidence and Prevalence of Schizophrenia and Other Psychotic Disorders in England'. Department of Health Policy Research Programme, University of Cambridge, King's College, London.

Kirsch, I. (2010) *The Emperor's New Drugs: Exploding the Antidepressant Myth*. New York: Basic Books.

Kitwood, T. (1997) *Dementia Reconsidered: The Person Comes First*. Buckingham: Open University Press.

Klein, R. (2010) *The New Politics of the NHS. From Creation to Reinvention*. Abingdon, Oxon: Radcliffe.

Knocker, S. (2012) *Perspectives on Ageing: Lesbians, Gay Men and Bisexuals*. York: Joseph Rowntree Foundation.

Krabbendam, L. (2005) 'Schizophrenia and urbanicity: environmental influence – conditional on genetic risk', *Schizophrenia Bulletin*, 31(4): 795–9.

Kramnaimuang, D., Judd, M. and King. T. (2012) 'Community epidemiology and environmental health risk from dioxin contamination in Paritutu', *Local Environment: The International Journal of Justice and Sustainability*: 1–13.

Krane, V. and Barak, K.S. (2012) 'Current events and teachable moments: creating dialog about transgender and intersex athletes', *Journal of Physical Education, Recreation and Dance*, 83(4): 38–43.

Ladd, P. (2003) *Understanding Deaf Culture: In Search of Deafhood*. Bristol: Channel View.

Lakasing, E. and Mirza, Z.A. (2009) 'The health of Britain's Polish migrants: a suitable case for history taking and examination', *British Journal of General Practice*, February: 138–9.

Laqueur, T. (1990) *Making Sex: Body and Gender from the Greeks to Freud*. Harvard: President and Fellows of Harvard College.

Laslett, P. (1989) *A Fresh Map of Life: The Emergence of the Third Age*. London: Weidenfeld and Nicolson.

Law, C. (2009) 'Life-course influences on children's futures', in H. Graham (ed.) *Understanding Health Inequalities*. Second edition. Maidenhead: Open University Press, McGraw-Hill Education, 25–47.

Law, J. (2006) *Big Pharma: Exposing the Global Healthcare Agenda*. New York: Carroll and Graf.

Lawrence, C. (1994) *Medicine in the Making of Modern Britain 1700–1920*. London: Routledge.

Lawton, J. (2000) *The Dying Process: Patients' Experiences of Palliative Care*. London: Routledge.

Laybourne, K. (1995) *The Evolution of British Social Policy and the Welfare State*. Edinburgh: Keele University Press.

Lievesley, N. (2009) *Ageism and Age Discrimination in Secondary Health Care in the United Kingdom. A Review from the Literature*. London: Centre for Policy on Ageing, Department of Health.

Light, D.W. (2003) 'Towards a new professionalism in medicine: quality, value and trust', *Tidsskr Nor Lægeforen*, 123.

Link, B.G. and Phelan, J.C. (2001) 'Conceptualizing Stigma', *Annual Review of Sociology* 27: 363–85.

Long, J., Hylton, K., Spracklen, K., Ratna, A. and Bailey, S. (2009) *Systematic Review of the Literature on Black and Minority Ethnic Communities in Sport and Physical Recreation*. Conducted for Sporting Equals and the Sports Council. Leeds: Carnegie Research Institute, Leeds Metropolitan University.

LSE Centre for Economic Performance's Mental Health Policy Group (2012) *How Mental Illness Loses Out in the NHS*. London: London School of Economics.

Lucas, A., Murray, E. and Kinra, S. (2013) 'Health beliefs of UK South Asians related to lifestyle diseases: a review of qualitative literature', *Journal of Obesity*, 2013: 1–12.

Luhrmann, T.M. (2010) 'The protest psychosis: how schizophrenia became a black disease' (review article), *Am J Psychiatry*, 167: 479–80.

Lumsden, K. (2010) 'Gendered performance in a male-dominated sub-culture: "Girl racers", car modification and the quest for modernity', *Sociological Research Online*, 15(3) 6 <www.socresonline.org.uk/15/3/6.html> 10.5153/sro.2123

Lupton, D. (2012) *Medicine as Culture: Illness, Disease and the Body in Western Societies*. Third edition. London: Sage.

Macdonald, B. with Rich, C. (2002) *Look Me in the Eye: Old Women, Ageing and Ageism*. San Francisco, CA: Spinsters Ink.

Macdonald, K. (1995) *The Sociology of the Professions*. London: Sage.

MacLean, A., Sweeting, H. and Hunt, K. (2010) '"Rules" for boys, "guidelines" for girls: gender differences in symptom reporting during childhood and adolescence', *Social Science & Medicine*, 70: 597–604.

Malik, K. (2009) *Strange Fruit: Why Both Sides are Wrong in the Race Debate*. Oxford: One World Publications.

Malterud, K. and Okkes, I. (1998) 'Gender differences in general practice consultations: methodological challenges in epidemiological research', *Family Practice*, 15(5): 404–10.

Marmot, M. and Wilkinson, R. (eds) (2009) *Social Determinants of Health*. Oxford: Oxford University Press.

Marmot, M., Allen, J., Goldblatt, P., Boyce, T., McNeish, D., Grady, M., Geddes, I. (2010) *Fair Society, Healthy Lives: The Marmot Review: Strategic Review of Health Inequalities in England Post-2010*. London: The Marmot Review.

Marongiu, A., Hope, V.D., Parry, J.V. and Ncube, F. (2012) 'Male IDUs who have sex with men In England, Wales and Northern Ireland: are they at greater risk of bloodborne virus infection and harm than those who only have sex with women?' *Sexually Transmitted Infections*, 88: 456–61.

Marshall, B. (2012) 'Medicalization and the refashioning of age-related limits on sexuality', *The Journal of Sex Research*, 49(4): 337–43.

Martin, J.S., Ummenhofer, W., Manser, T. And Spirig, R. (2010) 'Interprofessional collaboration among nurses and physicians: making a difference in patient outcome', *Swiss Medical Weekly*, 140: 1–12.

Marx, K. and Engels, F. (1848/2003) *The Communist Manifesto*. London: Bookmarks.

Mathur, R., Grundy, E., and Smeeth, L. (2013) *Availability and Use of UK Based Ethnicity Data for Health Research*. ESRC, National Centre for Research Methods.

McAndrew, S. and Warne, T (2004) 'Ignoring the evidence dictating practice: sexual orientation, suicidality and the dichotomy of the mental health nurse', *Journal of Mental Health Nursing*, 11(4): 428–34.

McCartney, G. (2011) 'Contribution of smoking-related and alcohol-related deaths to the gender gap in mortality: evidence from 30 European countries', *Tobacco Control*, 20: 166–68.

McCormick, J. with Clifton, J., Sachrajda, A., Cherti, M. and McDowell, E. (2009) *Getting on: Well-being in Later Life*. Institute for Public Policy Research.

McGrath, J., Saha, S., Welham, J., El Saadi, O., MacCauley, C. and Chant, D. (2004) 'A systematic review of the incidence of schizophrenia: the distribution of rates and the influence of sex, urbanicity, migrant status and methodology', *BMC Medicine*, 2(13).

McKeigue, P. (2001) 'Approaches to investigating the genetic basis of ethnic differences in disease risk', in H. Macbeth and P. Shetty (eds) *Health and Ethnicity*, London: Taylor and Francis: 113–32.

McKenzie, K. (2008) 'Urbanization, social capital and mental health', *Global Social Policy*, 8(3): 359–77.

McKeown, T. (1979) *The Role of Medicine: Dream, Mirage or Nemesis*. Second edition. Oxford: Blackwell Publishers.

McLaughlin, E. (2009) 'Community cohesion and national security: rethinking policing and race', in A. Bloch and J. Solomos (eds) *Race and Ethnicity in the Twenty-First Century*. Basingstoke, New York: Palgrave Macmillan, 93–111.

McLeod, J. (2013) 'Social stratification and inequality', in C.S. Aneshensel, J.C. Phelan and A. Bierman (eds) *Handbook of the Sociology of Mental Health*. Second edition. Springer Netherlands: 229–53.

McManus, S., Meltzer, H., Brugha, T., Bebbington, P. and Jenkins, R. (eds) (2009) *Adult Psychiatric Morbidity in England, 2007. Results of a Household Survey.* NHS Information Centre for Health and Social Care.

McMichael, A. J., Friel, S., Nyong, A. and Corvalan, C. (2008) 'Global environmental change and health: impacts, inequalities, and the health sector', *British Medical Journal*, January, 336: 191–4.

Mental Health Foundation (2012) website: www.mentalhealth.org.uk/help-information/mental-health-a-z/O/older-people/ [accessed 7 May 2013].

Middleton, S., Hancock, R., Kellard, K., Beckhelling, J., Phung, V. and Perren, K. (2007) *The Needs and Resources of Older People.* York: Joseph Rowntree Foundation.

Miles, R. and Brown, M. (2003) *Racism. Key Ideas.* Second edition. London: Routledge.

Milligan, M.S. and Neufeldt, A.H. (2001) 'The myth of asexuality: a survey of social and empirical evidence', *Sexuality and Disability*, 19(2): 91–109.

Millon, T. (2004) *Masters of the Mind: Exploring the Story of Mental Illness from Ancient Times to the New Millenium.* Chichester: John Wiley and Sons.

Millward, D. and Karlsen, S. (2011) *Tobacco Use Among Minority Ethnic Populations and Cessation Interventions.* A Race Equality Foundation Briefing Paper. London: Race Equality Foundation.

Minichiello, V., Browne, J. and Kendig, H. (2000) 'Perceptions and consequences of ageism: views of older people', *Ageing and Society*, 20: 253–78.

Moffatt, A. and Wilson, J.F. (2011) *The Scots. A Genetic Journey.* Edinburgh: Birlinn.

Moore, C. (2000) 'Sorting by sex', *American Scientist*, 88: 545–6.

Morgan, C., McKenzie, K. and Fearon, P. (eds) (2008) *Society and Psychosis.* Cambridge: Cambridge University Press.

Morgan, M., Calnan, M. and Manning, N. (1985) *Sociological Approaches to Health and Medicine.* London: Croom Helm.

Mossakowski, K.N. (2003) 'Copying with perceived discrimination: does ethnic identity protect mental health?' *Journal of Health and Social Behavior*, September, 44: 318–31.

Mottier, V. (2008) *Sexuality. A Very Short Introduction*. Oxford: Oxford University Press.

Moussavi, S., Chatterji, S., Tandon, A., Patel, V. and Ustun, B. (2007) 'Depression, chronic diseases, and decrements in health: results from the World Health Surveys', *The Lancet*, 370: 851–8.

Moynihan, R. (2010) 'Merging of marketing and medical science: female sexual dysfunction', *British Medical Journal*, 341:c5050.

Mulder, B.C., de Bruin, M., Schreurs, H. and van Emeijden, E.J.C. (2011) 'Stressors and resources mediate the association of socioeconomic position with health behaviours', *BMC Public Health*, 11: 798.

Myin-Germeys, I. and van Os, J. (2008) 'Adult adversity: Do early environment and genotype create lasting vulnerabilities for adult social adversity in psychosis?' in C. Morgan, K. McKenzie and P. Fearon (eds) *Society and Psychosis*. Cambridge: Cambridge University Press, 127–42.

Najman, J. (1980) 'Theories of disease causation and the concept of general susceptibility: a review', *Social Science and Medicine*, 14A: 231–7.

National Institute for Health and Clinical Excellence (2011) *Common Mental Health Disorders. Identification and Pathways to Care*. NICE clinical guideline 123. Developed by the National Collaborating Centre for Mental Health.

National Reporting and Learning System (2013) *Quarterly Data Workbook up to March 2012*. Available at: www.nrls.npsa.nhs.uk/resources/?entryid45=135152

Navarro, V. (1976) *Medicine Under Capitalism*. London: Croom Helm.

Nazroo, J. Y. (2010) 'Chapter Six: Health and health care', in A. Bloch and J. Solomos (eds) *Race and Ethnicity in the Twenty-First Century*. Basingstoke, New York: Palgrave Macmillan, 112–37.

Nettleton, S. (1995) *The Sociology of Health and Illness*. Cambridge: Polity.

Nettleton, S. (2004) 'The emergence of E-scaped medicine', *Sociology*, 38(4): 661–79.

Nettleton, S. (2006) *The Sociology of Health and Illness*. Second edition. Cambridge: Polity.

Nicholls, A. (2006) *Assessing the mental health needs of older people*. London: Social Care Institute for Excellence.

Nicholls, D.A. and Cheek, J. (2006) 'Physiotherapy and the shadow of prostitution: The Society of Trained Masseuses and the massage scandals of 1894', *Social Science and Medicine*, 62: 2336–348.

O'Donnell, C.A., Higgins, M., Chauhan, R. and Mullen, K. (2007) '"They think we're OK and we know we're not". A qualitative study of asylum seekers' access, knowledge and views to health care in the UK', *BMC Health Services Research*, 7: 75.

O'Reilly, D. and Reed, M. (2010) '"Leaderism": an evolution of managerialism in UK public service reform', *Public Administration*, 88(4): 960–78.

O'Riordan, K. (2012) 'The life of the gay gene: from hypothetical genetic marker to social reality', *Journal of Sex Research*, 49(4): 362–8.

Oakley, A. (1980) *Women Confined. Towards a Sociology of Childbirth.* Oxford: Martin Robertson.

Office for National Statistics (2010) *General Lifestyle Survey.* London: ONS.

Office for National Statistics (2010/2011) *Family Resources Survey.* London: ONS.

Office for National Statistics (2011a) *General Lifestyle Survey.* London: ONS.

Office for National Statistics (2011b) *Social Trends 41. Health.* London: ONS.

Office for National Statistics (2012a) *Intercensal Mortality Rates by NS-SEC, 2001–2010. Statistical Bulletin.* 24 April 2012.

Office for National Statistics (2012b) *2011 Census, Key Statistics for Local Authorities in England and Wales.* Released 11 December. London: ONS.

Office for National Statistics (2012c) *Older Workers in the Labour Market.* London: ONS.

Office for National Statistics (2012d) *Patterns of Pay: Results of the Annual Survey of Hours and Earnings 1997 to 2011.* February. London: ONS.

Office for National Statistics (2012e) *Labour Force Survey.* Quarter 2, 2012. London: ONS.

Office for National Statistics (2012f) *Life Opportunities Survey.* London: ONS.

Office for National Statistics (2013a) *Cohort Fertility, England and Wales, 2011.* London: ONS.

Office for National Statistics (2013b) *Alcohol-related Deaths in the United Kingdom, 2011.* London: ONS.

Office for National Statistics (2013c) *Suicides in the United Kingdom, 2011.* London: ONS.

Oliver, M. (1996) *Understanding Disability: From Theory to Practice.* London: Macmillan.

Ouwehand, C., de Ridder, D.T. and Bensing, J.M. (2009) 'Who can afford to look to the future? The relationship between socio-economic status and proactive coping', *European Journal of Public Health,* 19(4): 412–17.

Paechter, C. (2007) *Being Boys; Being Girls: Learning Masculinities and Femininities.* Maidenhead, Berkshire: McGraw Hill, Open University Press.

Parker, R. (2009) 'Sexuality, culture and society: shifting paradigms in sexuality research', *Culture, Health and Sexuality: An International Journal for Research, Intervention and Care,* 11(3): 251–66.

Parr, N.J. (2005)' Family background, schooling and childlessness in Australia', *Journal of Biosocial Science,* 37: 229–43.

Parsons, T. (1950) *The Social System.* Glencoe: Free Press.

Peen, J., Schoevers, R.A., Beekman, A.T. and Dekker, J. (2010) 'The current status of urban-rural differences in psychiatric disorders', *Acta Psychiatrica Scandinavica,* 121(2): 84–93.

Peterson, A. and Bunton, R. (1997) *Foucault, Health and Medicine.* London: Routledge.

Pickard, S. and Rogers, A. (2012) 'Knowing as practice: self-care in the case of chronic multi-morbidities', *Social Theory and Health,* 10(2): 101–20.

Pollock, A.M. (2010) 'Editorial: The Private Finance Initiative: The gift that goes on taking', *British Medical Journal,* 341: 1280–81.

Popay, J. and Jones, G. (1991) *Exploring the Sting in the Tail: Gender inequalities in health, domestic labour and socio-economic circumstances*. Thomas Coram Research Unit Working Paper. London: University of London.

Poundstone, K.E., Strathdee, S.A. and Celentano, D.D. (2004) 'The social epidemiology of Human Immunodeficiency Virus/Acquired Immunodeficiency Syndrome', *Epidemiologic Reviews*, 26: 22–35.

Powers, P. (2003) 'Empowerment as treatment and the role of health professionals', *Advances in Nursing Science*, 26(3): 227–37.

Prior, L. (1993) *The Social Organization of Mental Illness*. London: Sage.

Quart, A. (2003) *Branded: The Buying and Selling of Teenagers*. New York: Basic Books.

Rafalovich, A. (2013) 'Attention Deficit-Hyperactivity Disorder as the medicalization of childhood: challenges from and for sociology', *Sociology Compass*, 7(5): 343–54.

Razavi, S. (2011) 'Rethinking care in a development context: an introduction', *Development and Change*, 42(4): 873–903.

Reeve, J., Lloyd-Williams, M., Payne, S., and Dowrick, C. (2010) 'Revisiting biographical disruption: exploring individual embodied illness experience in people with terminal cancer', *Health (London)*, 14(2): 178–95.

Ridge, D. and Ziebland, S. (2012) 'Understanding depression through a "coming out" framework', *Sociology of Health and Illness*, 34(5): 730–45.

Ritzer, G. (1996) *The McDonaldization of Society*. Thousand Oaks, CA: Pine Forge Press.

Ritzer, G. (2010) *Globalization. A Basic Text*. Oxford: Wiley-Blackwell.

Rogers, A. and Pilgrim, D. (2010) *A Sociology of Mental Health and Illness*. Fourth edition. Maidenhead: Open University Press.

Rogoff, B. (2003). *The Cultural Nature of Human Development*. Oxford: Oxford University Press.

Rolfe, H. and Metcalf, H, (2009) *Recent Migration into Scotland: The Evidence Base*. National Institute of Economic and Social Research, Scottish Government Social Research.

Rosenfeld, J. (2010) '"The meaning of poverty" and contemporary quantitative poverty research', *The British Journal of Sociology*, 61 (issue supplement s1): 103–10.

Rosman, A., Rubel, P.G. and Weisgrau, M. (2009) *The Tapestry of Culture: An Introduction to Cultural Anthropology*. Ninth edition. Plymouth: Rowman and Littlefield.

Ross, C.A. and Goldner, E.M. (2009) 'Stigma, negative attitudes and discrimination towards mental illness within the nursing profession: a review of the literature', *Journal of Psychiatric and Mental Health Nursing* 16(6): 558–67.

Ross, C.E. and Mirowsky, J. (2013) 'The sense of personal control: social structural causes and emotional consequences', in C.S. Aneshensel, J.C. Phelan and A. Bierman (eds) *Handbook of the Sociology of Mental Health*. Second edition. Netherlands: Springer: 379–402.

Royal College of Nursing (RCN) (2005) *Lesbian, Gay, Bisexual and Transgender Patients or Clients. Guidance for Nursing Staff on Next-of-Kin Issues*. London: RCN.

Royal Society of Public Health (2005) 'The worried well: is health promotion to blame?' *Journal of the Royal Society for the Promotion of Public Health,* 125(2): 51.

Ryan, S. and Carr, A. (2010) 'Chapter Five: Applying the biospsychosocial model to the mManagement of rheumatic disease', in K. Dziedzic and A. Hammond (eds) *Rheumatology – Evidence-Based Practice for Physiotherapists and Occupational Therapists.* London, New York: Churchill Livingstone Elsevier: 63–75.

Saks, M. (2006) 'The alternatives to medicine', in D. Kelleher, J. Gabe and G. Williams (eds) *Challenging Medicine.* Second edition. London: Routledge, 85–103.

Sanders, T., Foster, N.E., Bishop, A. and Ong, B.N. (2013) 'Biopsychosocial care and the physiotherapy encounter: physiotherapists' accounts of back pain consultations', *BMC Musculoskeletal Disorders,*14: 65.

Sargent, M.G. (2005) *Biomedicine and the Human Condition: Challenges, Risks and Rewards.* Cambridge: Cambridge University Press.

Scambler, G. (2004) 'Reframing stigma: felt and enacted stigma and challenges to the sociology of chronic and disabling conditions', *Social Theory and Health,* 2: 29–46.

Scambler, G. (2008) 'Chapter Thirteen: Deviance, Sick Role and Stigma' in G. Scambler (ed.) *Sociology as Applied to Medicine.* Sixth edition. London: W. B. Saunders.

Scambler, G. (2009) 'Health-related Stigma', *Sociology of Health and Illness* 31(3): 441–55.

Scambler, G. (2011) 'Epilepsy, stigma and quality of life', *Neurology Asia,* 16 (Supplement 1): 35–6.

Scambler, G. and Paoli, F. (2008) 'Health work, female sex workers and HIV/AIDS: global and local dimensions of stigma and deviance as barriers to effective interventions', *Social Science and Medicine,* 66(8): 1848–62.

Scheff, T. (1966) *Being Mentally Ill: A Sociological Theory.* Chicago: Aldine.

Scheid, T.L. (2013) 'A decade of critique: notable books in the sociology of mental health and illness', Contemporary Sociology, 42(2): 177–83.

Schmid Mast, M., Sieverding, M., Esslen, M., Graber, K. and Jäncke, L. (2008) 'Masculinity causes speeding in young men', *Accident Analysis and Prevention,* 40(2): 840–2.

Scottish Dementia Working Group (2007) *What Disempowers Us – and what can be done.* Glasgow: Alzheimer Scotland.

Scull, A. (2009) *Hysteria: The Biography.* Volume 4 of the Oxford University Press Biographies of Diseases Series. Oxford University Press.

Seale, C.F. (2000) 'Changing patterns of death and dying', *Social Science and Medicine,* 51(6): 917–30.

Searle, E. (2002) 'Sexuality and people who are dying', in H. Heath and I. White (eds) (2002) *The Challenge of Sexuality in Health Care.* Oxford: Blackwell, 153–66.

Sedgwick, P. (1982) *Psychopolitics.* London: Pluto Press.

Sennett, R. (2008) *The Craftsman.* New Haven and London: Yale University Press.

Seymour, W. (1998) *Remaking the Body. Rehabilitation and Change.* London: Routledge.

Sharpley, M., Hutchinson, G., McKenzie, K. and Murray, R.M. (2001) 'Understanding the excess of psychosis among the African-Caribbean population in England', *British Journal of Psychiatry,* 178(40): 60–8.

Shaw, M., Davey Smith, G. and Dorling, D. (2005) 'Health inequalities and New Labour: how the promises compare with real progress', *British Medical Journal,* 330: 1016–21.

Sheridan, L. P. (2006) 'Islamophobia Pre-and Post-September 11th, 2001', *Journal of Interpersonal Violence,* 21(3): 317–36.

Shields, R. (2008) 'Homesick for Poland: Migrants' dreams in tatters'. *The Independent,* 24 August.

Singleton, N., Bumpstead, R., O'Brien, M., Lee, A. and Meltzer, H. (2001) *Psychiatric Morbidity Among Adults Living in Private Households, 2000.* London: HMSO.

Skeggs, B. (2009) 'Haunted by the spectre of judgement: respectability, value and affect in class relations', in K.P. Sveinsson (ed.) *Perspectives: Who Cares About the White Working Class?* London: Runnymede Trust: 36–44.

Smith, L. (2005) 'Psychology, classism and the poor: conspicuous by their absence', *American Psychologist,* 60(7): 687–96.

Smith, R.C., Fortin, A.H., Dwamena, F. and Frankel, R.M. (2013) An Evidence-Based Patient-Centred Method Makes the Biopsychosocial Model Scientific. *Patient Education and Counselling,* 91(3): 265–70.

Smolinksi, K. M. and Colón, Y. (2011) 'Palliative care with lesbian, gay, bisexual and transgender persons', in T. Altilio and S. Otis-Green (eds) *Oxford Textbook of Palliative Social Work.* Oxford: Oxford University Press: 379–86.

Spencer, N. (2008) *Health Consequences of Poverty for Children.* London: End Child Poverty.

Spencer, S., Ruhs, M., Anderson, B. and Rogaly, B. (2007) *The Experiences of Central and East European Migrants in the UK.* York: Joseph Rowntree Foundation.

Springer, K.W. and Mouzon, D.M. (2011) '"Macho men" and preventative health-care: implications for older men in different social classes', *Journal of Health and Social Behavior,* 52(2): 212–27.

Sproston, K. and Mindell, J. (2006) *Health Survey for England: The Health of Minority Ethnic Groups.* London: The Information Centre.

Stafford, M., Bécares, L. and Nazroo, J. (2010) 'Chapter Eleven: Racial discrimination and health: exploring the possible protective effects of ethnic density', in J. Stillwell and M. van Ham (eds) *Ethnicity and Integration.* Understanding Population Trends and Processes 3. Springer, 225–50.

Stiker, H. (2000) *A History of Disability.* (Corporealities: Discourses of Disability). Ann Arbor, MI: University of Michigan Press.

Stringhini, S., Sabia, S., Shipley, M., Brunner, E., Nabi, H., Kivimaki, M. and Singh-Manoux, A. (2010) 'Association of socioeconomic position with health behaviors and mortality', *The Journal of the American Medical Association,* 303(12): 1159–66.

Suglia, S.F., Duarte, C.S., Sandel, M.T. and Wright, R.J. (2010) 'Social and environmental stressors in the home and childhood asthma', *Journal of Epidemiology and Community Health,* 64: 636–42.

Synnott, A. (1993) *The Body Social. Symbolism, Self and Society.* London: Routledge.

Szasz, T. (1960) *The Myth of Mental Illness. Foundations of a Theory of Personal Conduct*. New York: Harper and Row.

Szasz, T. (2007) *Psychiatry's War on Criminal Responsiblity. In The Medicalization of Everyday Life. Selected Essays*. New York: Syracuse University Press.

Szreter, S. (1988) 'The importance of social intervention in Britain's mortality decline', *Social History of Medicine*, 1: 1–38.

Takács, J. (2004) 'The double life of Kertbeny', in G. Hekma (ed.) *Past and Present of Radical Sexual Politics*. Amsterdam: UvA-Mosse Foundation: 26–40.

Talairach-Vielmas, L. (2007) *Moulding the Female Body in Victorian Fairy Tales and Sensation Novels*. Aldershot, Hampshire: Ashgate.

Teghtsoonian, K. (2009) 'Depression and mental health in neoliberal times: a critical analysis of policy and discourse', *Social Science and Medicine*, 69: 28–35.

Thomas, B., Dorling, D. and Davey Smith, G. (2010) 'Inequalities in premature mortality in Britain: observational study from 1921 to 2007', *British Medical Journal* 341c3639: 1–6.

Thomas, C. (2010) 'Medical sociology and disability theory', in G. Scambler and S. Scambler (eds) (2010) *New Directions in the Sociology of Chronic and Disabling Conditions: Assaults on the Lifeworld*. Basingstoke, New York: Palgrave Macmillan.

Thomas, P. (2011) '"Mate crime": Ridicule, hostility and targeted attacks against disabled people', *Disability and Society*, 26(1): 107–11.

Thornicroft, G. (2006) *Shunned. Discrimination Against People with Mental Illness*. Oxford: Oxford University Press.

Thornicroft, G., Rose, D. and Kassam, A. (2007) 'Discrimination in health care against people with mental illness', *International Review of Psychiatry*, 19(2): 113–22.

Thurley, D. (2013) *State Pension Age – 2012 Onwards*. SN6546. London: Business and Transport Section, House of Commons.

Tiefer, L. (2010) 'Beyond the medical model of women's sexual problems: a campaign to resist the promotion of "female sexual dysfunction"', *Sexual and Relationship Therapy*, 25(2): 197–205.

Tillin, T., Forouhi, N.G., McKeigue, P.M. and Chaturvedi, N. (2006) 'The role of diabetes and components of the metabolic syndrome in stroke and coronary heart disease mortality in UK White and African-Caribbean populations', *Diabetes Care*, 29(9) September: 2127–9.

Timmermans, S. (2000) 'Social death as self-fulfilling prophecy: David Sudnow's *Passing On* revisited', in L. McKie and N. Watson (eds) *Organized Bodies. Policy, Institutions and Work*. London: Macmillan: 132–48.

Tomkins, L. and Eatough, V. (2012) 'Stop "helping" me! Identity, recognition and agency in the nexus of work and care', *Organization*: 1–19.

Townsend, P. (1979) *Poverty in the United Kingdom: A Survey of Household Resources and Standards of Living*. Berkeley, CA: University of California Press.

Townsend, P. (1981) 'The structured dependency of the elderly: a creation of social policy in the twentieth century', *Ageing and Society*, 1(1): 5–28.

Townsend, P., Whitehead, M. and Davidson, N. (1988) *Inequalities in Health: The Black Report: The Health Divide*. London: Penguin.

Traynor, M., Stone, K., Cook, H., Gould, D. and Maben, J. (2013) 'Disciplinary processes and the management of poor performance among UK nurses: bad apple or systemic failure? A scoping study', *Nursing Inquiry*: 1–8.

Trevena, P. (2009) *New Polish Migrants to the UK: A Synthesis of Existing Evidence*. Economic and Research Council, Centre for Population Change.

Tudor Hart, J. (1971) 'The inverse care law', *The Lancet*, 297 (7696): 405–12.

Tulle-Winton, E. (1999) 'Growing old and resistance: towards a cultural economy of old age?' *Ageing and Society*, 19: 281–99.

Tyler, I. (2008) '"Chav mum, chav scum": Class disgust in contemporary Britain', *Feminist Media Studies*, 8 (1): 17–34.

Urry, J. (2007) *Mobilities*. London: Polity.

Vaillant, N. and Wolff, F. (2012) 'On the reliability of self-reported health: evidence from Albanian data', *Journal of Epidemiology and Global Health*, 2: 83–98.

Van Hout, M. and Staniewicz, T. (2012) 'Roma and Irish traveller housing and health: a public health concern', *Critical Public Health*, 22(2): 193–207.

Varese, F., Smeets, F., Drukker, M., Lieverse, R., Lataster, T., Viechtbauer, W., Read, J., van Os, J. and Bentall, R.P. (2012) 'Childhood adversities increase the risk of psychosis: a meta-analysis of patient-control, prospective- and cross-sectional cohort studies', *Schizophrenia Bulletin*, 29 March 2012.

Victor, C., Scambler, S. and Bond, J. (2009) *The Social World of Older People, Understanding Loneliness and Social Isolation in Later Life*. Maidenhead: Open University Press.

Vincent, J.A. (2003) *Old Age*. Key Ideas Series. London: Routledge.

Vincent, J.A. (2006) 'Ageing contested: anti-ageing science and the cultural construction of old age', *Sociology*, 40: 681–98.

Vincent, J.A. (2009) 'Ageing, anti-ageing and anti-anti-ageing: who are the progressives in the debate on the future of human biological ageing?' *Medicine Studies*, 1: 197–208.

Wade, D.T. and Halligan, P.W. (2004) 'Do biomedical models of illness make for good healthcare systems', *British Medical Journal*, 329: 1398–401.

Wagemans, A., van Schrojenstein Lantman-de-Valk, H., Tuffrey-Wijne, I., Widdershoven, G. and Curfs, L. (2010) 'End-of-life decisions: an important theme in the care for people with intellectual disabilities', *Journal of Intellectual Disability Research*, 54(6): 516–24.

Wagner, K.S., Lawrence, J., Anderson, L., Yin, Z., Delpech, V., Chiodini, P.L., Redman, C. and Jones, J. (2013) 'Migrant health and infectious diseases in the UK: findings from the last ten years of surveillance', *Journal of Public Health*, March. Doi:10.1093/pubmed/fdt021.

Walters, K.L., Evans-Campbell, T., Simoni, J.M., Ronquillo, T. and Bhuyan, R. (2011) '"My spirit in my heart". Identity experiences and challenges among American Indian Two-Spirit women', in A. Pattatucci Aragón (ed.) *Challenging Lesbian Norms. Intersex, Transgender, Intersectional and Queer Perspectives*. London, New York: Routledge: 125–50.

Walters, K., Breeze, E., Wilkinson, P., Price, G.M., Bulpitt, C.J. and Fletcher, A. (2004) 'Local area deprivation and urban-rural differences in anxiety and depression among people older than 75 years in Britain', *American Journal of Public Health*, 94 (10): 1768–74.

Wang, J.L. (2004) 'Rural-urban differences in the prevalence of major depression and associated impairmen', *Social Psychiatry and Psychiatric Epidemiology*, 39: 19–25.

Wanless, D. (2002) *Securing our Future Health: Taking a Long-Term View: Final Report*. London: HM Treasury.

Warner, R. (2008) 'Social factors as a basis for treatment', in C. Morgan, K. McKenzie and P. Fearon (eds) *Society and Psychosis*. Cambridge: Cambridge University Press, 163–78.

Watt, G. (2004) 'What will the new genetic information do for us?' *Journal of Health Services Research and Policy*, 9(3): 186–8.

Watters, E. (2010) *Crazy Like Us. The Globalization of the American Psyche*. New York: Free Press.

Weber, J. and Wahl, J. (2006) 'Neurosurgical aspects of trepanations from neolithic time', *International Journal of Osteoarchaeology*, 16: 536–45.

Weber, M. (1976) *Economy and Society: An Outline of Interpretive Sociology* (2 vols). Berkeley, CA: University of California Press.

Weber, M. (edited by Roth, G. and Wittich, C.) (1978) *Economy and Society*. London, Berkeley, CA: University of California Press.

Weeks, J. (2010) *Sexuality*. Third edition. London: Routledge.

Wells, P. (2002) 'No sex please, I'm dying. A common myth explored', *European Journal of Palliative Care*, 9(3): 119–22.

Wenchao, J., Joyce, R., Phillips, D. and Sibieta, L. (2011) *Poverty and Inequality in the UK: 2011*. London: Institute for Fiscal Studies.

Wendell, S. (2001) 'Unhealthy disabled: treating chronic illness as disabilities', *Hypatia*, 16(4): 17–33.

White, P. (ed.) (2005) *Biopsychosocial Medicine. An Integrated Approach to Understanding Illness*. Oxford: Oxford University Press.

Whitley, R. (2011) 'Social defeat or social resistance? Reaction to fear of crime and violence among people with severe mental illness living in urban "recovery centres"', *Culture, Medicine and Psychiatry*, 35: 519–35.

Wilkinson, R. and Pickett, K. (2010) *The Spirit Level: Why More Equal Societies Almost Always Do Better*. Second edition. London: Allen Lane.

Williams, B., Copestake, P., Eversley, J. and Stafford, B. (2008) *Experiences and Expectations of Disabled People – Executive Summary. A research report for the Office for Disability Issues*. London: Office for Disability Issues, DWP.

Wilson, G. (2000) *Understanding Old Age*. London: Sage.

Wilton, T. (2000) *Sexualities in Health and Social Care*. Buckingham, Philadelphia: Open University Press.

Witz, A. (1992) *Professions and Patriarchy*. London: Routledge.

Witzig, R. (1996) 'The medicalisation of race: scientific legitimisation of a flawed social construct', *Annals of Internal Medicine*, 125: 675–9.

Wolf, N. (1991) *The Beauty Myth. How Images of Beauty are Used Against Women*. New York: William Morrow.

Wood, R., Sutton, M., Clark, D., McKeon, A. and Bain, M. (2006) 'Measuring inequalities in health: the case for healthy life expectancy', *Journal of Epidemiology and Community Health*, 60(12): 1089–92.

World Health Organization (2006). *Defining sexual health: Report of a technical consultation on sexual health, 28–31 January 2002*. Geneva: World Health Organization.

Wright Mills, C. (1959) *The Sociological Imagination*. Oxford: Oxford University Press.

WRVS (2011) *Gold Age Pensioners. Valuing the Socio-Economic Contribution of Older People in the UK*. Cardiff: WRVS.

Young Equals (2009) *Making the Case: Why Children Should be Protected from Age Discrimination and How it can be Done. Proposals for the Equality Bill*. London: Children's Rights Alliance for England.

Ziebland, S. and Wyke, S. (2012) 'Health and illness in a connected world: how might sharing experiences on the internet affect people's health?' *The Milbank Quarterly*, 90(2): 219–49.

Zimmerman, C. and Stöckl, H. (2012) *Human Trafficking*. Information Sheet. Understanding and Addressing Violence Against Women series. Geneva: World Health Organization.

Zola, I.K. (1972) 'Medicine as an institution of social control', in C. Cox and A. Mead (eds) (1975) *A Sociology of Medical Practice*. London: Collier-Macmillan, 170–85.

Zola, I. (1975) 'In the name of health and illness: on some socio-political consequences of medical influence', *Social Science and Medicine*, 9(2): 83–87.

Index

accountability, 164–166
Acheson Report, 48–49
activism, 118, 128–129, 135–136, *135*
Activities of Daily Living (ADL), 81
affective psychoses, 152
African Asians, 63
African Caribbeans, 63, 65, 69, 70–71,
    72–73, 150
Africans, 63, 65, 70
ageing
    health and, 79–83, *81*
    history of, 76–79
    implications for practice, 89
    interdependence and, 84
    life course approach and, 79–80
    material resources and, 52
    mental health and, 152
    overview, 75
    poverty and, 83–84
    society and, 87–88
    women and, 102
ageism, 77, 84–87, *85*
alcohol. *See* drinking
anaesthetics, 156
anatomy, 10
anorexia nervosa, 30, 142
anti-psychiatry movement, 145–146
antibiotics, 28
antidepressant medications, 148
antiseptics, 156
anxiety, 100, 143, 151
arthritis, 126
Asians, 61–62, 63
    See also Bangladeshis; Indians; Pakistanis
asthma, 79
asylum seekers, 64, 71
asylums, 124
Asylums (Goffman), 131
Atkinson, P., 132
Attention Deficit Hyperactivity Disorder
    (ADHD), 31

Bangladeshis, 63, 64, 69
barber surgeons, 156, *156*
barriers, 130
Beauty Myth, 101

binge drinking, 104
biographical disruption, 133–134
biomedicine (biomedical model)
    ageing and, 76
    challenges to, 11–12
    characteristics of, 9–11
    chronic illness and, 122–123, 124
    death and, 89
    definition of, 7
    disability and, 122–123, 124, 127–128
    gender and, 93, 105
    history of, 7–9, *20*, 40
    mental health and, 140, 141–142
    overview, 6–7
    physiotherapy and, 157
    sexuality and, 109
    sociological criticisms of, 13–14
biopsychosocial model, 15–18, 21
bipolar disorder, 152
birth control, 29–30
bisexual people, 114
    See also lesbian, gay, bisexual and transgender
        (LGBT) people
Black Africans, 63
Black Report, 48–49, 50
Blair Labour Government, 161–162
Blau, P.M., 163
body
    chronic illness and, 136–137
    disability and, 136–137
    as machine, 10, 13, 122–123
    mind and, 7–8, *8*, 10, 124
Body Mass Index (BMI), 33–34
breast cancer, 114
Breivik, A., 33
Brown, G.W., 151
bullying, 130
bureaucracy, 162–163, 164
Bury, M., 133

cancer, 104, 126, 133, 134
capitalism, 26–27, *27*, 40
cardiovascular disease, 27, 62
care, 128–129
census, 47, 61
Central Europeans, 63

cerebral palsy, 79, 102
charity, 123
Charmaz, K., 134, 135
childbirth, 27, 30, 99, 114
childhood diseases, 12
children and childhood
   disability and, 131
   health and, 79
   history of, 76, 78–79
   mental health and, 147, 150–151
Chinese, 63, 65
Christianity, 108–109
chronic illness
   biographical disruption and, 133–134
   body problems, 136–137
   history of, 123–125
   implications for practice, 137–138
   overview, 12, 122–123
   personal meaning and, 134–136
   socio-economic disadvantage and, 129–132
   in the UK, 125–127
chronic pain, 136–137
chronic pelvic pain (CPP), 17
chronic respiratory illness, 133
cirrhosis, 104
civil rights movement, 59
cochlear implants, 128
cohorts, 80
community care, 167
complementary and alternative medicine (CAM),
   19, 20–21, 36
compulsive eating, 142
The Condition of the English Working Class
   (Engels), 40–41
congenital malformation, 102
consumerism, 87, 148
contraception, 29–30
Cooper, M., 132, 133
coronary heart disease (CHD), 63, 66,
   102, 105
Courtenay, W.H., 103
Cubit, K., 86
cultural differences, 65–67
cultural resources (cultural capital), 50–51
Cumming, E., 78
cystic fibrosis, 79

Darr, A., 66
Darwin, C., 109
Davidson, R., 54
de la Rue, M., 86
Deaf community, 128
death and dying, 29, 88–89, 120
   See also mortality

dementia, 80, 81–82, 126
depression
   alcohol and, 104
   in Britain, 143
   ethnic minorities and, 62, 63
   incidence of, 142
   older people and, 82–83, 85
   social factors and, 149, 150
   women and, 100, 151
Descartes, R., 7–8, 8, 10
diabetes
   children and, 79
   ethnicity and, 62, 63, 67, 68, 68
   stigma and, 133
Diagnostic and Statistical Manual of Mental
   Disorders, 32, 110, 142
diarrhoeal diseases, 27
diet, 66
disability
   biographical disruption and, 133–134
   body problems, 136–137
   history of, 123–125
   implications for practice, 137–138
   medical and social models of, 127–129
   overview, 122–123
   personal meaning and, 134–136
   sexuality and, 120
   socio-economic disadvantage and, 129–132
   in the UK, 125–127
Disability Discrimination Act (2005), 126
disability studies, 134
disablism, 134, 135
discourse, 34
discrimination, 152–153
dopamine, 147
drapetomania, 58
drinking
   gender and, 104, 105
   mental health and, 152
   religion and, 66
   sexuality and, 114
Durkheim, É., 158
dyslexia, 32

East African Asians, 63
Eastern Europeans, 63
eating disorders, 95, 101
education, 130
electroconvulsive shock therapy, 141
emotion, 10–11
employment, 97, 130
empowerment, 168
Engel, G., 15
Engels, F., 40–41, 129

Enlightenment
  capitalism and, 26
  chronic illness and, 124
  disability and, 124
  gender and, 93
  health care and, 162
  medicine and, 8–9
  race and, 58
environmental justice movement,
  169–170
epilepsy, 132, 135–136
Equality Act (2010), 69–70, 84, 105
Essai sur l'homme (Descartes), 8
ethnicity and ethnic minorities
  in Britain, 61–62
  cultural differences and, 65–67
  definition of, 60–61
  genetic differences and, 64–65
  health benefits of, 72–73
  health differences related to, 62–64
  implications for practice, 73
  overview, 57
  race and, 59–61
  racism and, 69–72
  socio-economic factors and, 68–69
  See also migration
eugenics movement
  disability and, 124–125
  mental health and, 141
  Nazi Germany and, 59, 125
  overview, 35

female sexual dysfunction (FSD), 31–32
femininities, 92, 93, 95, 108
feminism, 145, 158–159
Fish, J., 114, 116
Foucault, M., 33, 34
Frank, A.W., 136, 137
Freud, S., 110, 151
Friedson, E., 158

Gaebler, T., 163
gay people. *See* homosexuality
gay rights movement, 110
gender
  definition of, 92
  health and, 97–104
  health care and, 158–159
  history of, 92–94
  implications for practice, 105
  inequality and, 96–97
  mental health and, 151–152
  overview, 91–92
  sexuality and, 108

gender *cont.*
  social construction of, 94–96
  See also women
gender sensitivity, 105
gender stereotyping, 105
General Household/Lifestyle Survey, 47
genetic differences, 64–65
genetic tests, 35
germ theory, 11
gerontology, 78
Gliddon, G.R., 58
globalization, 168–170
gloves, 111–112
Goffman, E., 117, 125, 131, 152, 167
Gull, W., 30

haemoglobin disorders, 72–73
hallucinations, 34
hate crime, 130, 131
health
  ageing and, 79–83, 81
  class and, 42–44, 50
  ethnic minorities and, 62–64
  ethnicity and, 62–64, 72–73
  gender and, 97–104
  globalization and, 168–170
  LGBT people and, 113–116
  new approaches to, 19–21, 20
  older people and, 80–83, 81
  as socially constructed, 14
health care
  accountability and, 164–166
  bureaucracy and, 162–163, 164
  community care and, 167
  globalization and, 168–170
  history of, 156–157
  implications for practice, 170
  lay people and, 18–19, 18, 36, 164
  managerialism and, 162, 163–164
  mental health and, 153
  negative effects of, 28–29
  overview, 155
  participation and, 168
  power and, 36–37
  sexuality and, 114–116
  women and, 101–102
Health Care Assistants, 159–160
health care professionals, 157–160
hegemonic masculinity, 95–96, 102–103
Henderson, J., 86
Henry, W.E., 78
hepatitis, 114
heterosexism, 116–117
Hillman, A., 165–166

Hindus, 66, 72–73, 76
HIV/AIDS
  biographical disruption and, 133
  Disability Discrimination Act and, 126
  GBT men and, 114
  in the majority world, 27
  migrants and, 67–68
  stigma and, 117–118
  women and, 105
Holm-Denoma, J.M., 95
Holmes, T.H., 151
homosexuality
  gender norms and, 95
  medicalization of, 32, 109, 110,
    112–113
  origin of term, 109
  religion and, 116
  See also lesbian, gay, bisexual and transgender
    (LGBT) people
housing, 71
Human Papillomavirus (HPV), 113–114
human trafficking, 169
Hunt, R., 114
hyperactivity, 31
hyperkinetic syndrome, 31
hypertensive disease, 63, 104
hysteria, 93, 142

iatrogenesis, 28
identity
  definition of, 72
  disability and, 131
  sexuality and, 107, 112–113
Illich, I., 28–29, 30, 36
Indians
  health and, 62–63, 64, 69
  smoking and, 66
  termination of pregnancy and,
    72–73
industrialism, 124
inequality, 41–42, 96–97
infantilization, 77
infectious diseases, 11, 12, 27, 126
injury, 79
institutional racism, 69–72
insulin coma therapy, 141
inter-marriage, 61
interdependence, 84
internet, 36–37, 119, 119
interprofessional education (IPE),
    166, 166
intersex, 91, 92, 113, 115
intimate partner violence, 100–101
Irish people, 62, 66

Irish traveller communities, 71
Is Mental Illess a Myth? (Szasz), 145–146

Johnson, T., 158

Knocker, S., 115
Koedijck, I., 156
Koh, L.C., 86

labelling, 145
labour market, 71
language barriers, 69
Laslett, P., 83
Lawrence, C., 69
lay epidemiology, 169–170
lay people
  definition of, 18
  health care and, 18–19, 18, 36, 164
  prevention and, 17
learning disabilities, 32, 126–127,
    130, 132
lesbian, gay, bisexual and transgender (LGBT)
    people, 113–116
lesbianism, 109, 110, 114
life course, 80
life course approach, 79–80
life expectancy, 98
Limits to Medicine (Illich), 28
liver cirrhosis, 66
living wills, 88–89
loss of self, 134
lung infections, 27

majority world
  capitalism and, 27
  definition of, 12
  infectious diseases in, 12
  race and, 59
malaria, 27, 65, 67–68
malnutrition, 14, 27
managerialism, 162, 163–164
Marmot, M., 48–49, 51
Martinez, F., 136
Marx, K., 26, 40–41, 162
masculinities, 92, 93, 95, 108
masturbation, 109
mate crime, 131
material resources, 51–53
measles, 14
mechanical metaphor, 10
media, 148–149
Medical Act (1858), 157
medical gaze, 34
medical tourism, 169

medicalization
  of childbirth, 30, 158
  of death, 88–89
  definition of, 30
  of homosexuality, 32, 109, 110,
    112–113
  of mental illness, 148
  overview, 29–33
  of sexuality, 112–113, 119
meningitis, 79
men's health, 102–104
mental health
  adversity across the life course and,
    150–151
  biological factors in, 144,
    147–149
  in Britain, 142–143, **143**
  history of, 141–142
  implications for practice, 153
  older people and, 83, 85
  overview, 140
  sexuality and, 113–114, 117
  social factors in, 144,
    149–150
  as socially constructed, 144–147
  stigma and, 141, 152–153
migration, 61, 67–68, 149, 150
mind, 7–8, *8*, 10, 124
Mojola, S.A., 118
monasteries, 131
morbidity
  gender and, 97–99
  social class and, 47–49, *47*, *48*
mortality
  gender and, 98–99
  learning disabilities and,
    126–127
  social class and, 44–45, *45*, **46**
motor neurone disease, 133
Moyle, W., 86
Muff March, *101*
multiple sclerosis, 126, 133
Muslim women, 66
Muslims, 66, 71, 72–73

National Assistance Act (1948), 125
National Health Service, 160
National Insurance, 160
National Statistics Socio-economic Classification
    system (NE-SEC), **43**, 44
Nazi Germany, 59, 125
Nazroo, J. Y., 67
neoliberalism, 160–162
Nettleton, S., 10, 100

norms
  definition of, 16
  gender and, 103
  sexuality and, 108
  social factors and, 15–16
Nott, C., *58*
Nurses Registration Act (1919), 157

obesity, 33–34, 79
oestrogen, 105, 152
Office of National Statistics, 47
Old Age Pensions, 77
older people
  chronic illness and, 126
  health and, 80–83, *81*
  poverty and, 83–84
  sexuality and, 120
Oliver, M., 128
Osborne, D., 163

Pakistanis, 63, 64, 66, 72–73
Parkinson's disease, 126
Parsons, T., 25, 29
part-time work, 97
participation, 168
party, 41
patient-centred medicine, 36, 168
personal meaning, 134–136
personhood, 77, 134
pharmaceutical industry, 148
physiology, 1
physiotherapy, 157
Piaget, J., 78
Pickett, K., 53
Polish migrants, 62, 63
Poor Laws, 77, 123
Post Traumatic Stress Disorder, 141
poverty
  children and, 79
  class and, 49
  ethnic minorities and, 63
  gender and, 97
  as health hazard, 14, 27
  mental health and, 149
  old age and, 83–84
  women and, 97, 100
power
  authority and, 24
  capitalism and, 26–27
  definition of, 24
  discourse and, 34
  health care and, 36–37
  implications for practice, 37
  medical gaze and, 34

power *cont.*
    overview, 23–24
    risk and, 35
    sick role and, 25–26, 29
    surveillance and, 33, 35
prefrontal lobotomy, 141
pregnancy, 27, 72–73
premature birth, 102
prevention, 17
Prior, L., 167
prisons, 124, 131
psychiatric hospitals, 131
psychiatry, 32–33, 141–142
psychology, 1
psychosis, 63, 70–71, 147, 151
psychosocial factors
    definiton of, 16
    social class and, 53–55
public health system, 26

Quechua community (Peru), 144–145

race, 58–61
racism, 59, 69–72
Rahe, R.H., 151
recreational drugs, 114
refugees, 64
Registrar General, 42–44, **43**,
    45, 96
rehabilitation, 128–129
reliability, 47–48
religion, 66, 72–73, 107, 116
remission society, 137
retirement, 77
rheumatoid arthritis, 133
risk, 35
Ritalin, 31
Robinson, A., 86
Roma traveller communities, 71

salutogenesis, 17, 18
Scambler, G., 132, 134, 135
schizophrenia
    African Caribbeans and, 70
    causes of, 147
    discourse and, 34
    neurological research and, 142
    social factors and, 149, 150
Scottish Dementia Working group, 82
screening programmes, 35
Second World War, 12, 94
self-care and self-diagnosis, 28–29, 36
self-harm, 101, 142
self-starvation, 30

senescence, 76
sex and sexuality
    celebration of, 118–120, *119*
    vs. gender, 94
    health and, 113–116
    heterosexism and, 116–117
    history of, 108–110
    implications for practice, 120
    overview, 107–108
    social construction of, 110–113
    stigma and, 114, 117–118
sex trafficking, 169
sexology, 109
sexual violence, 100
Sexually Transmitted Diseases (STDs), 113
Seymour, W., 129
Shameless (tv series), *55*
Shipman, H., 164
sick role, 25–26, 29
sickle cell disorders, 64, 65
sign language, 128
Sikhs, 66, 72–73
smoking, 52–53, 65–66, 104–105, 114
social capital, 54–55, 72
social class
    cultural resources and, 50–51
    definiton of, 40
    disability and, 124–125
    gender and, 96
    health and, 42–44, 50
    history of, 40–41
    implications for practice, 55–56
    inequality and, 41–42
    material resources and, 51–53
    mental health and, 149
    morbidity and, 47–49, *47*, *48*
    mortality and, 44–45, *45*, *46*
    overview, 39–40
    poverty and, 49
    psychosocial factors and, 53–55
social construction
    definition of, 60
    gender and, 94–96
    mental health and, 144–147
    race and, 60
    sexuality and, 110–113
social control, 26, 145, 158
social determinants of health, 37
social factors, 1–2, 15–16, 25
social gerontology, 78
social model of disability, 128–129
Society of Trained Masseuses, 157
socio-economic disadvantage, 129–131
socio-economic factors, 68–69, 96

socio-economic status, 44
sociological imagination, 2
sociology
    biomedicine and, 13–14
    definition of, 1
South Asians, 66
the state/states, 41, 42, 161
status, 41, 76, 92
stigma
    disability and, 131–132, 134
    learning disabilities and, 32
    mental health and, 141, 152–153
    sexuality and, 114, 117–118, *117*
Stigma (Goffman), 117, 131
stress, 71, 147
stroke, 63, 80, 126, 133
Sudden Infant Death Syndrome (SIDS), 32, 102
suicide, 63, 114, 152
surgery, 156
surveillance, 33, 35
Synnott, A., 9
Szasz, T., 145–146, 152

Tay-Sachs disease, 64–65
termination of pregnancy, 72–73
Thalidomide, 12
Thatcher Conservative Government, 161
Thomas, P., 134
total institutions, 124
Townsend, P., 78
tranquillizers, 142, 148
transgendered people, 93, 95, 113, 114
    See also lesbian, gay, bisexual and transgender
        (LGBT) people
trauma, 70, 151
trepanation, 141
tuberculosis (TB), 14, 27, 67–68, 98
Twigg, J., 111–112

Two-Spirits, 92
Types of Mankind (Nott and Gliddon), *58*

urbanicity, 149–150
US civil rights movement, *59*

violence, 131, 148–149, 152

Watt, G., 35
Weber, M., 41, 42, 162–163
Whitehead Report, 48–49
Wilkinson, R., 53
women
    ageing and, 102
    anorexia nervosa and, 30
    biomedicine and, 14
    birth control and, 29–30
    chronic pelvic pain and, 17
    depression and, 100, 151
    drinking and, 105
    female sexual dysfunction and, 31–32
    health care and, 158–159
    higher education and, 14
    mental health and, 151–152
    poverty and, 97, 100
    psychiatry and, 145–146
    sexuality and, 109
    smoking and, 52–53
    status and, 76, 92
    See also gender
women's health, 99–102
    See also childbirth
women's movement, 110
workhouses, 77, 124
World Health Organization (WHO),
    107–108

Zola, I., 29–30, 32, 131